THE CARE OF WOUNDS
A GUIDE FOR NURSES

SECOND EDITION

CAROL DEALEY BSc (Hons), RGN, RCNT, Pg Dip

Research Fellow
University Hospital Birmingham NHS Trust, and
School of Health Sciences
University of Birmingham

Blackwell
Science

© 1994, 1999 by
Blackwell Science Ltd
Editorial Offices:
Osney Mead, Oxford OX2 0EL
25 John Street, London WC1N 2BL
23 Ainslie Place, Edinburgh EH3 6AJ
350 Main Street, Malden
  MA 02148 5018, USA
54 University Street, Carlton
  Victoria 3053, Australia
10, rue Casimir Delavigne
  75006 Paris, France

Other Editorial Offices:

Blackwell Wissenschafts-Verlag GmbH
Kurfürstendamm 57
10707 Berlin, Germany

Blackwell Science KK
MG Kodenmacho Building
7–10 Kodenmacho Nihombashi
Chuo-ku, Tokyo 104, Japan

The right of the Author to be identified as the
Author of this Work has been asserted in
accordance with the Copyright, Designs and
Patents Act 1988.

First published 1994
Reprinted 1995, 1996
Second edition published 1999
Reprinted 2000

Set in 10/12 pt Souvenir
by DP Photosetting, Aylesbury, Bucks
Printed and bound in Great Britain by
MPG Books Ltd, Bodmin, Cornwall

The Blackwell Science logo is a
trade mark of Blackwell Science Ltd,
registered at the United Kingdom
Trade Marks Registry

DISTRIBUTORS

Marston Book Services Ltd
PO Box 269
Abingdon
Oxon OX14 4YN
(Orders: Tel: 01235 465500
       Fax 01235 465555)

USA
Blackwell Science, Inc.
Commerce Place
350 Main Street
Malden, MA 02148 5018
(Orders: Tel: 800 759 6102
                781 388 8250
         Fax: 781 388 8255)

Canada
Login Brothers Book Company
324 Saulteaux Crescent
Winnipeg, Manitoba R3J 3T2
(Orders: Tel: 204 837 2987
         Fax: 204 837 3116)

Australia
Blackwell Science Pty Ltd
54 University Street
Carlton, Victoria 3053
(Orders: Tel: 03 9347 0300
         Fax: 03 9347 5001)

A catalogue record for this title
is available from the British Library

ISBN 0-632-05237-6

Library of Congress
Cataloging-in-Publication Data
is available

For further information on
Blackwell Science, visit our website:
www.blackwell-science.com

Contents

Preface

In preparing this second edition of *The Care of Wounds* I have been interested to see that the principles that guided me in writing the original book have not greatly changed. In some areas there has been little further research and in others there has been much to consider. The management of wounds becomes increasingly complex with the constantly expanding range of wound management products and technologies. The concept of clinical effectiveness is very important and I have added an additional chapter on this topic. At all times I have tried to inform the reader of what is available, whilst at the same time recognising the need for a pragmatic approach to care in everyday practice.

I would like to thank all those who have encouraged me with their kind remarks about the original book. I hope that this edition will continue to meet the needs of all those who care for patients with wounds.

Carol Dealey

Chapter 1
The Physiology of Wound Healing

Wound healing is a highly complex process. It is important that the nurse has an understanding of the physiological processes involved for several reasons:

(1) An understanding of normal physiology makes it possible to recognise the abnormal.
(2) Recognition of the stages of healing allows the selection of appropriate dressings.
(3) Understanding of the requirements of the healing process means that appropriate nutrition can, as far as is possible, be given to the patient.

1.1 INTRODUCTION

Any damage leading to a break in the continuity of the skin can be called a wound. There are several causes of wounding:

- traumatic – mechanical, chemical, physical
- intentional – surgery
- ischaemia – e.g. arterial leg ulcer
- pressure – e.g. pressure sore

In both traumatic and intentional injury there is rupture of the blood vessels which results in bleeding, followed by clot formation. In wounds caused by ischaemia or pressure the blood supply is disrupted by local occlusion of the microcirculation. Tissue necrosis follows and results in ulcer formation, possibly with a necrotic eschar or scab.

Wounds in the skin, or deeper, have been labelled in various ways. Some of them can be described as follows:

(1) Partial- and full-thickness wounds
  - A partial-thickness wound is one where some of the dermis remains and there are shafts of hair follicles or sweat glands.
  - In a full-thickness wound all the dermis is destroyed and deeper layers may also be involved.
(2) Healing by first and second intention
  This was first described by Hippocrates around 350 BC.
  - Healing by first intention is when there is no tissue loss and the skin edges are held in apposition to each other, such as a sutured wound.
  - Healing by second intention means a wound where there has been tissue loss and the skin edges are far apart, such as a leg ulcer.

(3) Open and closed wounds
    ● These are the same as healing by second and first intention respectively.

1.2 WOUND HEALING

The wound healing process consists of a series of highly complex interdependent and overlapping stages. These stages have been given a variety of names. They are described here as:

● inflammation
● reconstruction
● epithelialisation
● maturation

The stages last for variable lengths of time. Any stage may be prolonged because of local factors such as ischaemia or lack of nutrients. The factors which can delay healing are discussed in more detail in Chapter 2.

1.3 INFLAMMATION

The inflammatory response is a non-specific local reaction to tissue damage and/or bacterial invasion. It is an important part of the body's defence mechanisms and is an essential part of the healing process. The signs of inflammation were first described by Celsus in the first century AD as redness, heat, pain and swelling. The factors causing them are shown in Table 1.1.

    When there is traumatic or intentional injury which causes damage to the blood vessels the first response is to stop the bleeding. This is achieved by a combination of factors. Firstly, by vasoconstriction which reduces the blood flow. Also by the release of a plasma protein called von Willebrand factor from both endothelial cells and platelets, resulting in platelet aggregation and formation of a platelet plug. The third factor is the initiation of the clotting cascade and the development of a fibrin clot to reinforce the platelet plug.

Table 1.1 The signs of inflammation.

Signs and symptoms	Physiological rationale
Redness	Vasodilation results in large amount of blood in the area.
Heat	Large amount of warm blood and heat energy produced by metabolic reactions.
Swelling	Vasodilation and leakage of fluid into the wound area.
Pain	May be caused by damage to nerve ends, activation of the kinin system, pressure of fluid in the tissues or the presence of enzymes, such as prostaglandins, which cause chemical irritation.

Hageman factor (factor XII in the clotting cascade) triggers both the complement and kinin systems. The complement system consists of plasma proteins which are inactive precursors. When activated, there is a cascade effect which leads to the release of histamine and serotonin from the mast cells and results in vasodilation and increased capillary permeability. The complement system also assists in attracting neutrophils to the wound. The complement molecule, C3b, acts as an opsonin. That is, it assists in binding neutrophils to bacteria. Five of the proteins activated during the cascade process form the membrane attack complex which has the ability to directly destroy bacteria.

The effect of the complement system is enhanced by the kinin system which, through a series of steps, activates kininogen to bradykinin. Kinins attract neutrophils to the wound, enhance phagocytosis and stimulate the sensory nerve endings. The apparent delay in feeling pain after injury is explained by the short time lag taken for the kinin system to be activated.

As the capillaries dilate and become more permeable, there is a flow of fluid into the injured tissues. This fluid then becomes the 'inflammatory exudate' and contains plasma proteins, antibodies, erythrocytes, leucocytes and platelets. As well as being involved in clot formation, platelets also release fibronectin and growth factors called platelet-derived growth factor (PDGF) and transforming growth factor alpha and beta (TGFα and TGFβ). Their role is to promote cell migration and growth at the wound site.

Growth factors are a sub-class of cytokines, proteins that are used for cellular communication (Greenhalgh, 1996). The particular role of growth factors is to stimulate cell proliferation. There are a number of growth factors involved in the healing process, they are listed in Table 1.2. Some growth factors have been isolated and used as a treatment for chronic wounds. This will be discussed in more detail in Chapter 4.

Table 1.2 Growth factors involved in the healing process.

Growth factor	Action
Platelet-derived growth factor PDGF	Chemotactic for neutrophils, fibroblasts and, possibly, monocytes. Encourages proliferation of fibroblasts.
Transforming growth factor alpha TGFα	Stimulates angiogenesis.
Transforming growth factor beta TGFβ	Chemotactic for monocytes (macrophages). Encourages angiogenesis. Regulates inflammation.
Fibroblast growth factor FGF	Stimulates fibroblast proliferation and angiogenesis.
Epidermal growth factor EGF	Stimulates the proliferation and migration of epithelial cells.
Insulin-like growth factors IGF-I, IGF-II	Promote protein synthesis and fibroblast proliferation. Work in combination with other growth factors.

The first leucocyte to arrive at the wound is the neutrophil. Wagner (1985) has described the role of fibronectin in relation to neutrophils. It attracts neutrophils to the wound site, a process known as chemotaxis. Neutrophils squeeze through the capillary walls into the tissues by diapedesis, again this ability is enhanced by fibronectin. Within about an hour of the inflammatory response being initiated, neutrophils can be found at the wound site. They arrive in large numbers, their role being to phagocytose bacteria by engulfing and destroying them. Neutrophils decay after phogocytosis as they are unable to regenerate the enzymes required for this process. As the numbers of bacteria decline, so too do the numbers of neutrophils.

TGFβ attracts monocytes to the wound. Once in the tissues they are known as macrophages. Fibronectin binds on to the surface receptors on the cells promoting diapedesis and phagocytosis. Macrophages are larger than neutrophils and so are able to phagocytose larger particles, such as necrotic debris, as well as bacteria. The lifespan of the neutrophil can be a few hours or a few days. When they die they are also phagocytosed by the macrophages. Oxygen is required for this activity and if the partial pressure falls below 30 mmHg (mercury) then phagocytosis capability is reduced (Cherry *et al.*, 1995).

T lymphocytes also migrate into the wound, although in smaller numbers than macrophages (Martin & Muir, 1990). They influence macrophage phagocytic activity by the production of several macrophage regulating factors. They also produce colony stimulating factors which encourage the macrophage to produce a range of enzymes and cytokines. One such substance is prostaglandin which maintains vasodilation and capillary permeability. It can be produced on demand to prolong the inflammatory response if required. However, macrophages are also instrumental in promoting the transition from inflammation to the reconstruction phase of healing.

Inflammation lasts about 4–5 days. It requires both energy and nutritional resources. In large wounds the requirements may be considerable. If this stage is prolonged by irritation to the wound, such as infection, foreign body or damage caused by the dressing, it can be debilitating to the patient as well as delay healing.

1.4 RECONSTRUCTION

The reconstruction phase is characterised by the development of granulation tissue. It consists of a loose matrix of fibrin, fibronectin, collagen and hyaluronic acid and other glycosaminoglycans. Within this matrix can be found macrophages and fibroblasts and the newly formed blood vessels. Macrophages play a major role in this phase of healing, as shown in Fig. 1.1. They produce PDGF and fibroblast growth factor (FGF) which are chemotactic to fibroblasts, attracting them to the wound and stimulating them to divide and later to produce collagen fibres. Fibronectin also seems to play a role in enhancing fibroblast activity (Orgill & Demling, 1988). Collagen has been seen in a new wound as early as the second day. Collagen fibres are made up of chains of amino acids in a triple helix formation. There are a number of different types of collagen characterised by different formations of

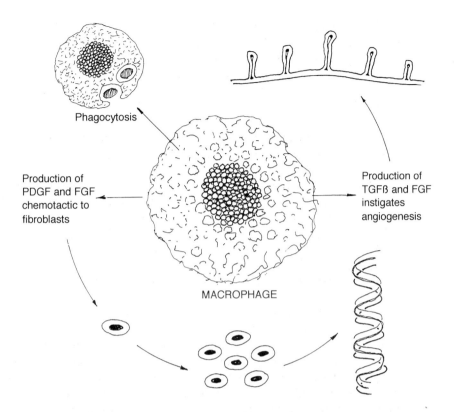

Phagocytosis

Production of
PDGF and FGF
chemotactic to
fibroblasts

Production of
TGFß and FGF
instigates
angiogenesis

MACROPHAGE

Fig. 1.1 The role of the macrophage.

amino acids. Type III is present in the healing wound in greater proportions than would normally be found in skin. Over time, this proportion reduces in favour of higher levels of type I collagen.

The activity of fibroblasts depends on the local oxygen supply. If the tissues are poorly vascularised the wound will not heal well. The wound surface has a relatively low oxygen tension, encouraging the macrophages to produce TGFß and FGF which instigates the process of angiogenesis, the growth of new blood vessels. Undamaged capillaries beneath the wound sprout buds which grow towards the surface and loop over and back to the capillary. The loops form a network within the wound supplying oxygen and nutrients.

Some fibroblasts have a further role. They are specialised fibroblasts known as myofibroblasts (Gabbiani *et al.*, 1973), which have a contractile apparatus, similar to that in smooth muscle cells, which causes contraction of the wound. Contraction may start at around the fifth or sixth day. It considerably reduces the surface area of open wounds. Irvin (1987) suggests that contraction could be responsible for as much as 40–80% of the closure. It is certainly of considerable importance in large cavity wounds. However, in wounds with a large surface area such as burns, contraction may lead to contractures.

In wounds healing by first intention, little can be seen of this stage of healing. But in those healing by second intention, the wound can be seen to be filled with granulation tissue. Figure 1.2 demonstrates the microscopic view of the macrophages forming the advance guard, clearing the wound cavity. They are followed by capillary buds growing towards the areas of low oxygen tension in the wound.

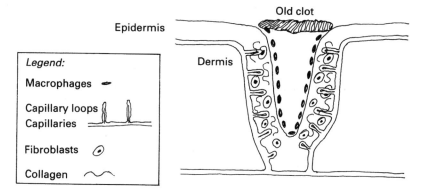

Fig. 1.2 The process of reconstruction.

As the wound fills with new tissue and a capillary network is formed, the numbers of macrophages and fibroblasts gradually reduce. This stage may have started before the inflammation stage is completed and prolonged inflammation can result in excessive granulation with hypertrophic scarring. The length of time needed for reconstruction depends on the type and size of wound, but may be about 24 days for wounds healing by first intention.

1.5 EPITHELIALISATION

This describes the phase in which the wound is covered with epithelial cells. Macrophages release epidermal growth factor (EGF) which stimulates both the proliferation and migration of epithelial cells. Keratinocytes at the wound margins and around hair follicle remnants synthesise fibronectin which forms a temporary matrix along which the cells migrate. The cells move over the wound surface in a leap-frog fashion, the first cell remaining on the wound surface and forming a new basement membrane. When cells meet, either in the centre of the wound, forming islets of cells, or at the margin, they stop. This is known as contact inhibition. Epithelial cells only move over viable tissue and require a moist environment (Winter, 1962). In sutured wounds, epithelial cells also migrate along the suture tracks. They are either pulled out with the sutures, or gradually disappear.

This phase commences as early as the second day in closed wounds. However, in open wounds it is necessary for the wound cavity to be filled with granulation tissue before epithelialisation can commence. There is a very variable time span for this stage.

1.6 MATURATION

During maturation the wound becomes less vascularised as there is a reduction in the need to bring cells to the wound site. The collagen fibres are reorganised so that, instead of being laid down in a random fashion, they lie at right angles to the wound margins. The scar tissue present is gradually remodelled and becomes comparable to normal tissue after a long period of time. The scar gradually flattens to a thin white line. This may take up to a year in closed wounds and very much longer in open wounds.

Tensile strength gradually increases. This is a way of describing the ability of the wound to resist rupture or dehiscence. Forester *et al.* (1969) found that at ten days an apparently well-healed surgical incision has little strength. During maturation it increases so that by three months the tensile strength is 50% that of normal tissue. Further work by Forester *et al.* (1970) compared surgical incisions where the skin edges were held together by tape with those where sutures were used. The findings showed that, when tape was used, the wounds regained 90% strength of normal tissue, whereas sutured wounds only regained 70% strength.

1.7 IMPAIRED WOUND HEALING

Although the majority of wounds heal without problem, impaired healing may sometimes occur. Some of the different types of impaired healing are described here. Their management will be discussed elsewhere.

1.7.1 Hypertrophic scars

Hypertrophic scars occur when there is an extreme fibrous tissue response during the healing process resulting in excessive deposition of collagen and a thick wound scar (Munro, 1995). Hypertrophic scars are more common after traumatic injury, especially large burns. They occur shortly after the injury or surgery and remain limited to the area of the injury. They will generally flatten out with time – about one to two years.

1.7.2 Keloids

Keloids are similar to hypertrophic scars in that they are also the result of an excessive fibrous response. The difference is that keloids take some time to form and may occur years after the initial injury. They can range in size from small papules to large pendulous growths (Munro, 1995). Keloids more commonly occur in individuals aged between 10 and 30 years (Cosman *et al.*, 1961) and in those with a darker skin (Placik & Lewis, 1992). Unfortunately, unlike hypertrophic scars, keloids do not gradually flatten out.

1.7.3 Contractures

Wound contraction is part of the normal healing process, but occasionally contraction will continue after re-epithelialisation has occurred resulting in scar contraction (Tredget *et al.*, 1997). Engrav *et al.* (1987) describe how this type of scar contracture can result in joint contracture with subsequent loss of mobility, functional loss, delay in return to work and a poor cosmetic result. Plate 1 shows contractures developing in a leg wound in an infant. There is potential here for both a poor cosmetic result and problems as the child grows which may result in a need for surgery.

1.7.4 Acute to chronic wounds

Chronic wounds may be called chronic because their underlying aetiology makes healing a very long process. A very good example is the venous leg ulcer. However, some chronic wounds may have originally been acute wounds which have failed to heal over a long period of time, perhaps years. The initial factor delaying healing may have been related to infection or local irritation, perhaps caused by a suture. Once these problems have been resolved, the wound still fails to heal, causing considerable misery to the patient.

The differences between acute and chronic wounds are still imperfectly understood. However, recent work by Phillips *et al.* (1998) may shed some light on the problem. They used cultured fibroblasts from human neonatal foreskin as a plated laboratory model and treated them with either chronic wound fluid (CWF) or bovine serum albumen (the control). They found that CWF inhibited the growth of the fibroblasts quite dramatically. The researchers concluded that this study gave some indication of how the microenvironment of a chronic wound has a negative effect on the healing wound. Further work is required to identify the factors responsible for this inhibition of the healing process.

1.8 CONCLUSION

This chapter has described 'normal' physiology. However, not all wounds heal without complication or delay. Many factors can affect the healing process. These factors will be considered in more detail in Chapter 2.

It is also important to recognise that although great strides have been made in the last ten to twenty years in the understanding of the healing process, it is still incompletely understood. No doubt, there will be further progress in the next few years.

FURTHER READING

Vander, A., Sherman, J., Luciano, D. (1998) *Human Physiology*, 7th edn. McGraw-Hill Companies Inc., Boston.

REFERENCES

Cherry, G.W., Hughes, M.N.A., Kingsnorth, A.N., Arnold, F.W. (1995) Wound healing, in (eds) Morris, P.J., Malt, R.A., *Oxford Textbook of Surgery*. Oxford University Press, Oxford.

Cosman, B., Crikelair, G.F., Ju, M.C. *et al.* (1961) The surgical treatment of keloids. *Plastic & Reconstructive Surgery*, **27**, 335–358.

Engrav, L.H., Covey, M.H., Dutcher, K.D. *et al.* (1987) Impairment, time out of school and time out of work after burns. *Plastic & Reconstructive Surgery*, **79**, 927.

Forester, J.C., Zederfeldt, B.H., Hunt, T.K. (1969) A bioengineering approach to the healing wound. *Journal of Surgical Research*, **9**, 207.

Forester, J.C., Zederfeldt, B.H., Hunt, T.K. (1970) Tape-closed and sutured wounds: a comparison by tensiometry and scanning electron microscope. *British Journal of Surgery*, **57**, 729.

Gabbiani, G., Hajno, G., Ryan, G.B. (1973) The fibroblast as a contractile cell: the myofibroblast, in (eds) Kulonen, E., Pikkarainen, J., *The Biology of the Fibroblast*. Academic Press, London.

Greenhalgh, D. (1996) The role of growth factors in wound healing. *Journal of Trauma*, **41** (1), 159–167.

Irvin, T.T. (1987) The principles of wound healing, *Surgery*, **1**, 1112–1115.

Martin, C.W., Muir, I.F.K. (1990) The role of lymphocytes in wound healing. *British Journal of Plastic Surgery*, **43**, 655–662.

Munro, K.J.G. (1995) Hypertrophic and keloid scars. *Journal of Wound Care*, **4** (3), 143–148.

Orgill, D., Demling, R.H. (1988) Current concepts and approaches to wound healing. *Critical Care Medicine*, **16** (9), 899–908.

Phillips, T.J., Al-Amoudi, H.O., Leverkus, M., Park, H-Y. (1998) Effect of chronic wound fluid on fibroblasts. *Journal of Wound Care*, **7** (10), 527–532.

Placik, O., Lewis, V.L. (1992) Immunological associations of keloids. *Surgery, Gynaecology & Obstetrics*, **175**, 185–193.

Tredget, E.E., Nedelec, B., Scott, P.G., Ghahary, A. (1997) Hypertrophic scars, keloids and contractures. *Surgical Clinics of North America*, **77** (3), 701–730.

Wagner, B.M. (1985) Wound healing revisited: fibronectin and company. *Human Pathology*, **16** (11), 1081.

Winter, G.D. (1962) Formation of the scab and the rate of epithelialisation of superficial wounds in the skin of the domestic pig. *Nature*, **193**, 293–294.

Chapter 2
The Management of Patients with Wounds

2.1 INTRODUCTION

This chapter looks at assessment of the patient with a wound and how appropriate care may be planned and evaluated. When caring for patients with wounds – of all types – it is important to adopt a holistic approach to patient care. There are many factors that can affect the healing process; if they are taken into account when taking a history and assessing the patient it may be possible to mitigate some of the effects. Nursing intervention is not able to resolve every problem, for example, age. Where nursing intervention can be effective, appropriate strategies are suggested.

A model of nursing provides a useful framework for assessing patients. The 'Activities of Living' is the model which has been selected to discuss the factors which can affect healing. However, although this model is very good when considering physical aspects of care, attention must also be given to psychological and spiritual care as the three are inextricably linked.

2.2 PHYSICAL CARE

2.2.1 Maintaining a safe environment

Disruption of a safe environment may be responsible for causing wounds, for example, accidents on the road or in the home. Factors within the environment may also affect healing.

Infection

Systemic infection affects healing as the wound has to compete with any infection for white cells and nutrients. Healing may not take place until after the body has dealt with the infection. Systemic infection is frequently associated with pyrexia. Pyrexia causes an increase in the metabolic rate, thus increasing catabolism or tissue breakdown.

All wounds are contaminated with bacteria, especially open wounds. This does not affect healing. However, clinical infection will certainly do so. Infection prolongs the inflammatory stage of healing as the cells combat the large numbers of bacteria. It also appears to inhibit the ability of fibroblasts to produce collagen (Senter & Pringle, 1985).

Infection in a burn wound increases the metabolic rate and thereby increases the time of negative nitrogen balance. Kinney (1977) has shown that there may be a loss of 20–30% of the initial body weight in the presence of major sepsis. Infection also causes pain which raises the metabolic rate (Arturson, 1978).

There have been several major studies of surgical wound infection rates, including those of Cruse and Foord (1973, 1980), Bibby *et al.* (1986) and Emmerson *et al.* (1996). These studies, especially that of Cruse and Foord, have highlighted factors which may predispose the patient to wound infection. It should be noted that the infection rates are usually compared with the expected infection rate of 1.5% for clean surgery. These factors include the following.

Age It has been found that patients over 65 years are six times more likely to develop an infection in a clean surgical wound than a child under 14 years (Cruse & Foord, 1973). Mishriki *et al.* (1990) found a significantly higher incidence of wound infection in patients over the age of 55 years. Moro *et al.* (1996) used logistical regression to identify factors associated with increased risk of surgical wound infection. They found that age greater than 85 years was a significant factor.

Build/weight for height Obesity increases clean wound infection rate to 13.5% (Cruse & Foord, 1973). Martens *et al.* (1995) found obesity to be a significant factor in wound infection following Caesarian section. These findings are supported by Moro *et al.* (1996), who found obesity to be a significant factor for infection in a wide range of surgical cases, and also by He *et al.* (1994) and Birkmeyer *et al.* (1998). Researchers in these latter two studies found a significantly higher incidence of sternal wound infection following bilateral internal mammary artery grafting and coronary artery bypass surgery respectively.

Nutritional status Poor nutrition increases the infection risk. McPhee *et al.* (1998) found preoperative protein depletion to be a significant factor for wound infection in patients undergoing spinal surgery. (See also Eating and drinking; Section 2.2.4)

Diabetes The management of diabetic patients undergoing surgery must be carefully monitored. Surgery can cause de-stabilisation which increases the risk of infection. In turn, infection can also affect the diabetic state. Hyperglycaemia affects the body's defence mechanism by impairing the response of white cells – neutrophils in particular. Cruse and Foord (1973) found a clean wound infection rate of 10.7% in diabetic patients. Borger *et al.* (1998) found diabetes to be a predictor of deep sternal wound infection for patients undergoing cardiac surgery.

Special risks Irradiation, steroids, and immunosuppressive drugs cause greatly increased infection rates (Bibby *et al.*, 1986). Chmell and Schwartz (1996) found that preoperative chemotherapy was a significant factor in wound infection following musculoskeletal sarcoma resections.

Length of preoperative stay   The longer the stay in hospital, the more chance there is that the patient's skin will become colonised by bacteria against which the patient has no resistance. Cruse and Foord (1980) found that the clean wound infection rate increased from 1.2% for a one-day preoperative stay to 2.1% for seven days and to 3.4% for more than 14 days.

Bed occupancy   Occupancy of more than 25 beds in an open ward increases wound infection (Bibby *et al.*, 1986).

Shave   It is impossible to carry out a shave without causing injury to the skin. Bacteria flourish and multiply rapidly in these minute cuts. The clean wound infection rate was found to be 2.5% in shaved patients compared with 1.7% for those who had had their pubic hair clipped and 0.9% for those who were not shaved (Cruse & Foord, 1980). Mishriki *et al.* (1990) and Moro *et al.* (1996) also found shaving to be a significant factor in the development of infection. Mishriki *et al.* suggest that this is particularly so when contaminated and dirty procedures are undertaken and bacteria are shed on the skin. It is generally recommended that if a patient needs to be shaved preoperatively, it should be done just prior to surgery.

Type of surgery   Infection rates are much higher in some types of surgery than others. This is discussed in more detail in Chapter 6. The appearance of infected wounds will be discussed in Chapter 3.

The elderly

Elderly people have an increased incidence of underlying disease. Some may directly affect the healing process. Others may cause a level of disability which can affect the patient's ability to maintain safe standards of hygiene, thus increasing the risk of infection.

Socioeconomic problems

Poor housing may not only cause hazards such as badly lit stairs, but other problems – damp or rodent infestation – which make it difficult to maintain cleanliness. This predisposes to disease as well as increasing the risk of infection.

● *Nursing assessment* ●

(1)   Infection: (a)   identify those at risk (see Table 2.1)
                   (b)   assess wound (see Chapter 3)
                   (c)   monitor temperature regularly.
(2)   The elderly: evidence of relevant underlying disease?
(3)   Socioeconomic problems: relevant if a patient with a chronic wound is to be cared for at home.

Table 2.1   Infection risk factors.

General factors	
Age	Very young or very old.
Nutrition	Emaciated; thin; obese; dehydrated.
Mobility	Limited; immobile; temporary; permanent.
Mental state	Confused; depressed; senile.
Incontinence	Urine; faeces; temporary; permanent.
General health	Weak; debilitated.
General hygiene	Dependence; mouth/teeth; skin.
Local factors	
Oedema	Pulmonary; ascites; effusion.
Ischaemia	Thrombus; embolus; necrosis.
Skin lesions	Trauma; burns; ulceration.
Foreign body	Accidental; planned.
Invasive procedures	
Cannulation	Peripheral; central; parenteral.
Catheterisation	Intermittent; closed; drainage; irrigation.
Surgery	Wound; wound drainage; colostomy; implant.
Intubation	Endobronchial suction; ventilation; humidification.
Drugs	
	Cytotoxics; antibiotics; steroids.
Diseases	
	Carcinoma; leukaemia; aplastic anaemia; severe anaemia; diabetes. Liver disease; renal disease; transplantation; AIDS.

Based on Bowell (1992)

● *Nursing interventions* ●

Problem: Actual/potential risk of infection
Goal: Prevention or early detection

The prevention of infection is the responsibility of all healthcare professionals. There are both general and specific measures which can be taken. Most health authorities have infection control policies which provide guidelines both for the prevention of infection and to reduce the risk of cross infection. The Infection Control Team, especially the Infection Control Nurse, can give advice and support.

Much has been written on the prevention of infection. Altemeier *et al.* (1984) provided guidelines on the prevention of infection in surgical patients. They cover such diverse topics as hospital design, housekeeping techniques, the health of the operating personnel, preparation of the patient, methods of sterilisation and more besides. Ayliffe *et al.* (1982) suggested general methods for the management and prevention of hospital-acquired infection, again covering a wide range of topics. Horton (1993) described a strategy for improving the knowledge base of all members of the multidisciplinary team with respect to infection control.

The spread of infection is mostly by people from people. Thus, the simplest and most effective measure to prevent infection is good handwashing. A review by Larson and Kretzer of the period 1984–1994 found that researchers consistently reported that whilst the action of handwashing was carried out mostly at the appropriate times, the methods used were ineffective (Larson & Kretzer, 1995). Gould (1992) also supports this view, but she suggests that there has been a failure to consider the reality of the situation in the clinical area. One example cited is that compliance is unlikely if the designated cleanser makes hands sore. Taylor (1978) produced recommendations for handwashing that ensured that all parts of the hands would be washed. They are still advocated today. The guidelines produced by Taylor identify three different types of handwashing. They include:

Social handwashing   Before the medicine round, before and after eating, when hands are obviously dirty, after going to the toilet and after patient contact.

Antiseptic handwashing   Beginning and end of a shift, before and after aseptic procedures, after handling bedpans and urinals, entering and leaving high-risk areas.

Surgical handwashing   Before all surgical procedures.

Identification of patients at risk of infection means that appropriate measures can be taken. Some particularly vulnerable patients may need extra measures. These may include the use of a single room with a positive pressure filtered air system, providing protective isolation, prophylactic drugs or special operating techniques such as a Charnley Howarth tent for orthopaedic procedures.

● *Evaluation* ●

Careful monitoring of vulnerable patients is essential. Monitoring a patient's temperature is a useful means of evaluation as a rise in temperature is often the first indication of infection. The use of clinical audit will identify areas where cross-infection may be a regular problem.

2.2.2 Communicating

The art of communicating is essential to nursing. It involves listening and identifying problems and anxieties as well as giving explanations. Failure to recognise stress or to involve the patient adequately in understanding care can affect wound healing.

Stress and anxiety

Lazarus and Averill (1972) stated that 'anxiety results when a person is unable to fully comprehend the world around him'. This could be considered in relation to ill health. A further quotation from Frankenhaeuser (1967) adds to this: 'Information is necessary for comprehension, but the perception of this information can be modified by the expectations of the subject'. Many nurses will have seen patients who have not heard or have misunderstood what has been said to them because of their degree of anxiety.

Admission to hospital, whether planned or unplanned can be a very stressful experience. Stress has a physiological effect. Stimulated by the release of adrenalin, a primary biochemical change in stress is an increased secretion of adrenocorticotrophic hormone (ACTH), which stimulates production of adrenal cortex hormones. In particular, ACTH regulates production of glucocorticoids, cortisol and hydrocortisone. Glucocorticoids cause the breakdown of body stores to glucose, raising the blood sugar. They cause a reduction in the mobility of granulocytes and macrophages, impeding their migration to the wound. In effect this suppresses the immune system and reduces the inflammatory response. Glucocorticoids also increase protein breakdown and nitrogen excretion which inhibits the regeneration of endothelial cells and delays collagen synthesis. There would seem to be an increased risk of wound infection in a very anxious patient. It has been shown that a reduction of anxiety caused a significant decrease in the incidence of postoperative wound infection (Boore, 1978). Kiecolt-Glaser and colleagues have researched the effects of psychological stress on 13 women and found it significantly slowed the rate of healing when compared with a group matched for sex, age and income (Kiecolt-Glaser *et al.*, 1995).

● *Nursing assessment* ●

Zigmond and Snaith (1983) have designed a simple questionnaire which identifies the degree of stress being suffered. It can be filled in by patients (see Fig. 2.1). They reported most patients found it simple to use and were enthusiastic about the concept.

The HAD score comprises a series of questions with a choice of answers using a ✓ box. Examples of some of the questions are given below.

I feel tense or 'wound up'

Most of the time	☐
A lot of the time	☐
Time to time, occasionally	☐
Not at all	☐

Worrying thoughts go through my mind

A great deal of the time	☐
A lot of the time	☐
From time to time, but not too often	☐
Only occasionally	☐

I can enjoy a good book or radio or TV programme

Often	☐
Sometimes	☐
Not often	☐
Very seldom	☐

Fig. 2.1 The HAD score.

● *Nursing interventions* ●

Problem: Anxiety related to hospital admission.
Goal: Patients will be able to express their specific anxieties.

Many patients find their admission to hospital a very anxious time. Volicer and Bohannon (1975) found that lack of communication increased stress. Dale (1993) considered that little notice had been taken of this finding. The initial assessment should provide both information and an opportunity for patients to ask questions and express their feelings and concerns. Not all patients will feel able to discuss their anxieties immediately. It may be an ongoing process of building up a relationship over a period of time. A study by Wilkinson (1992a) of cancer patients on six wards in two hospitals showed that most patients desired open communication with those caring for them. Unfortunately, her study found that some nurses blocked communication with patients because they saw it as the doctor's role or they found it too distressing. Some felt they would like to talk truthfully with their patients, but lacked the skills to do so. Certainly, every nurse should cultivate the art of listening.

Wilkinson (1992b) considered that an inability to communicate adequately with patients resulted in nurses failing to identify all the patients' physical problems let alone their psychological ones. Morrison and Burnard (1989) suggest that nurses will work more efficiently if they communicate effectively.

Active listening is not a very safe occupation. The consequences may be emotionally painful to the nurse because of the difficult questions that may be asked. Many may feel inadequate or too inexperienced. Koshy (1989) describes active listening as 'the process of receiving and assimilating ideas and information from verbal and non-verbal messages and responding appropriately'. Tschudin (1991) emphasises the importance of not making assumptions: it is too easy for nurses to assume that they not only know the problem, but also have the answers for dealing with it.

● *Evaluation* ●

Repetition of the assessment will enable the nurse to identify any reduction in stress levels.

Problem: Anxiety related to surgery.
Goal: Patient's anxiety will be reduced by adequate preoperative preparation.

There is a much greater awareness of the importance of providing good preoperative information. A Department of Health circular (1990) makes it clear that all patients have the right to understand their treatment and the risks involved. Janis (1958) found that stress levels were as high in patients undergoing what could be classed minor surgery as in those having major surgery. Smith (1992) described how a lack of understanding of the convalescent period following surgery also caused considerable anxiety. Beddows (1997) found that preoperative information, both oral and written, plus an opportunity to have questions answered significantly reduced anxiety in comparison with a control group who received standard information.

The role of the nurse is to ensure that each patient receives appropriate pre-operative information about the surgery and about what to expect in the post-operative period. Radcliffe (1993) has considered how a suitable strategy can be implemented. She suggests that oral information is reinforced with written leaflets which can be a source of reference to both patients and relatives.

● *Evaluation* ●

The patient should be able to describe the likely course of events in the perio-perative and postoperative period.

Alternative therapies

Some alternative therapies have been successfully used to assist patients in reducing anxiety. Marshall (1991) described how aromatherapy and relaxation techniques were being used to reduce stress in dermatology patients. Dossey (1991) used case studies to discuss the benefits of guided imagery. This is a method of relaxation which encourages patients to use their imagination first to identify the health problem and then to visualise how the treatment will work effectively – this may involve favourite scenes, music or other audiotapes. Ultimately patients have to visualise themselves in the final healed state. Patients should use this technique over a period of time, such as for two weeks prior to surgery, for it to be effective. It is easy to dismiss such a concept as 'mumbo-jumbo' because it is alien to many healthcare professionals. Holden-Lund (1988) randomly allocated cholecystectomy patients to either guided imagery or period of quiet. Those receiving guided imagery had significantly lower anxiety levels, cortisol levels and surgical wound erythema compared with the control group.

Therapeutic touch has been used in the USA for a number of years to reduce anxiety levels. Heidt (1981) used matched patient groups in a cardiovascular unit to receive either therapeutic touch, casual touch or no touch. Those receiving thera-peutic touch had significantly lower levels of anxiety compared with the other groups.

Pain

Pain and anxiety are closely related because pain can increase anxiety and anxiety increase pain. Blaylock (1968) suggested that this was because the nervous response to pain and to anxiety is the same. Hayward (1975) showed that pre-operative information to reduce anxiety resulted in less postoperative pain. Fear of pain can cause much anxiety to patients. Pracek *et al.* (1995) found that procedural pain experienced by burn patients in the early stages of their admission could be a causal factor in their ability to adjust after discharge. The greater the pain levels, the poorer the adjustment.

There is a wealth of evidence that lack of adequate pain control is common. Carr (1997) described four barriers to effective pain control:

(1) *Lack of knowledge and inappropriate attitudes of healthcare professionals.*
A large study by the Royal College of Surgeons and College of Anaesthetists (1990) on pain after surgery found that nurses had insufficient commitment to providing adequate pain control and a lack of relevant knowledge; as a result up to 75% of patients experience moderate to severe postoperative pain. Field (1996) found that nurses consistently underestimated the pain suffered by their patients. Closs (1992) found that patients' sleep was disturbed by pain. In his study of 100 surgical patients, 49 said the pain was worse at night.

It is not only patients undergoing surgery that experience unrelieved pain. A study was carried out by Chan *et al.* (1990). They studied the prevalence of chronic pain in diabetic patients. They found that chronic pain was more common in those suffering from diabetes than in those who did not. The pain was most commonly reported to be in the lower limbs. The researchers noted that there seemed to be little recognition of the problem or facilities to help resolve it. Hitchcock *et al.* (1994) surveyed over 200 individuals who suffered from chronic pain. They found that on average the respondents suffered pain 80% of the time, and 50% of the respondents reported that their prescribed analgesia was inadequate.

(2) *Patients expect pain.*

(3) *Patients may minimise their pain.*
Yates *et al.* (1995) studied older patients in long-term residential care. They found that these patients were resigned to having pain and expected that they would just have to tolerate it. They also reported being reluctant to discuss their pain for fear of being labelled a complainer. Carr and Thomas (1997) found similar results when they interviewed postoperative patients. Ward *et al.* (1996) discussed cancer patients' perceptions of pain and noted that many feared that they would become addicted to their analgesia. Others do not complain because they believe that 'good' patients should not complain. Also, pain to the cancer patient indicates further progression of the disease and the patient may be reluctant to report increased pain.

(4) *The organisation may inhibit the provision of good pain relief.*
Fagerhaugh and Strauss (1977) considered the organisational structure within which pain management takes place. They suggested that workload in the clinical area, lack of accountability and the complexity of the nurse–patient relationship were all factors that resulted in poor pain management. The acute pain team can play a major role in improving the standards of assessment and organisation of analgesia which results in improved pain control (Harmer & Davies, 1998). However, there can also be problems. Carr and Thomas (1997) suggest that ward nurses still fail to recognise their responsibilities for pain management and may abdicate their role to the pain management team. They also found that nurses tended to assume that 'high tech' equipment, such as patient-controlled analgesia (PCA), automatically abolished pain and therefore pain assessment was not necessary.

Parsons (1992) gives an overview of studies of cultural aspects of pain and concludes that definitions of pain by both the sufferer and carer are shaped by cultural beliefs. In some cultures free expression of feelings of pain is expected whereas in others it is unacceptable. There needs to be recognition of these cultural differences in order to manage pain successfully.

● *Nursing assessment* ●

Holzman and Turk (1986) describe pain as a unique experience for each individual. It therefore follows that only the patient can describe its presence and severity. Pedley (1996) reviewed some of the assessment tools that have been developed. She recommends the use of a visual analogue scale (see Fig. 2.2). However, elderly people do not always find such a concept easy to use. Verbal analogue scales may be more suitable. This type of scale uses descriptions ranging from no pain through mild, moderate and severe to unbearable pain. Simons and Malaber (1995) considered the problem of patients who cannot communicate by speech, and developed a method of assessing behaviour and body language.

● *Nursing interventions* ●

> *Problem: Inadequate pain control.*
> *Goal: Patients will be able to express feelings of comfort and relief from pain.*

Pain management is a big topic and can only be addressed briefly here. Modern systems of drug delivery such as slow-release drugs, or intravenous pumps, provide constant pain relief that is more effective than the use of injections, which have a bolus effect. Spinal infusion has been found work well in a small group of terminally ill patients for whom other methods failed (Hicks *et al.*, 1994).

Music has been used as a distraction therapy to help reduce a patient's perception of pain in the immediate postoperative period (Taylor *et al.*, 1998). Relaxation has been successfully used as a technique to reduce pain in cancer patients (Sloman *et al.*, 1994) and in older men undergoing hip replacement (Parsons, 1994). Other strategies may be used to assist in pain relief. Measures such as turning, lifting or massage may be very comforting. Simple aids such as a bed cradle to reduce the weight of the bedclothes can be very effective.

● *Evaluation* ●

Regular use of a pain chart allows constant evaluation of the effectiveness of pain relief.

Motivation and education

Stronge (1984) suggests that involving patients in the care or protection of their wounds promotes healing. Logically, careful explanation of the importance of diet or appropriate exercise can only improve the rate of healing. A positive attitude to healing by the nurse has a significant effect on the outlook of the patient. Fernie and Dornan (1976) found it improved the healing of pressure sores.

The education of surgical patients has been studied extensively in the USA and the UK (Cook, 1984). It has been used to reduce the length of hospital admission following surgery and thus costs. A corollary can be drawn: improved recovery implies wound healing without complication.

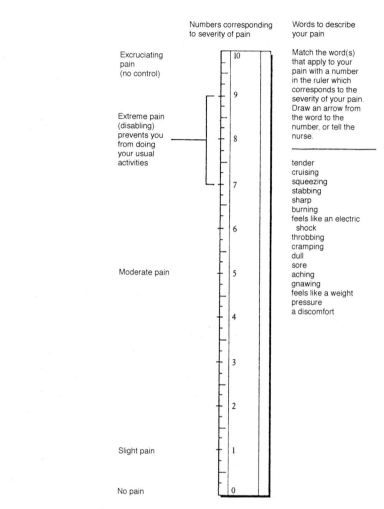

Fig. 2.2 A pain chart
(from Bourbonnais, 1981).

Nyatanga (1997) has reviewed psychosocial theories of noncompliance and divided them into the following categories:

- *Perceptual theory*: people interpret the world based on what they already know. They may have pre-existing theories about their treatment.

- *Value clarification*: patients may consider the choices in relation to their treatment and choose whether to comply. An example would be the man choosing not to give up smoking despite knowing it increases his risk of leg amputation.

- *Attribution theory*: this relates to the locus of control. Patients who feel in control of their treatment or who see a link between their treatment and the healing of their wound are more likely to be compliant.

- *Cultural theories*: all individuals have a cultural understanding of their wound, its meaning and the treatment. This may lead them to decide not to follow all the treatment requirements, such as not wishing to take analgesia.

- *The health belief model*: patients may choose to engage in health-related behaviour if they believe that the benefits in terms of health gain outweigh the costs. For example, a leg ulcer patient may choose to wear a four layer bandage which she finds hot and uncomfortable because she believes that it will heal her ulcer.

● *Nursing assessment* ●

Simple questioning can determine the level of relevant knowledge that a patient possesses.

● *Nursing interventions* ●

Problem: A lack of understanding of the care needed to promote wound healing.
Goal: Patients will be capable of self-caring and able to explain their plan of care.

In the climate of early discharge from hospital, many patients will return home with a wound that still requires dressing. If it is practicable, it is helpful to teach patients to undertake their own dressings. Monitoring and supervision by the district nurse or practice nurse would still be necessary. A planned education programme using short-term goals is the most effective. Information about allied care such as diet or exercise can also be incorporated into the programme. Patients with chronic wounds should be given information about their causes and possible prevention.

Some patients will have little motivation to carry on the plan of care once they have been discharged from hospital. Recognition of the reasons for the lack of motivation and good communication with the community staff may be of some help. A few patients will still fail to respond. It is necessary to accept that every patient has the right to choose not to comply with the care recommended by the healthcare team.

● *Evaluation* ●

The ability of the patient to undertake management of the wound will provide adequate evaluation of the effectiveness of the nursing care.

2.2.3 Breathing

A good blood supply to the wound and an adequate supply of oxygen are an essential part of healing. Various factors can adversely affect this.

Age

The circulation is less efficient in the elderly. This may be associated with disease.

Cardiovascular disease

Impaired circulation reduces tissue perfusion. This slows healing and increases the risk of infection. Although tissue hypoxia stimulates angiogenesis (Knighton et al., 1981), it impairs all metabolism and overall growth rate. Peripheral vascular disease is often a complication of diabetes mellitus. It has a detrimental effect on the healing of wounds on the lower limbs and may even be a precipitating factor.

Smoking causes vasoconstriction and is associated with Buerger's Disease, a condition causing intermittent claudication and gangrene. Moseley et al. (1978) suggested that smoking also interfered with the proliferation of erythrocytes, thereby reducing the available oxygen. A review of the effects of smoking on wound healing by Siana et al. (1992) found that nicotine affected macrophage activity and reduced epithelialisation and wound contraction. Jorgensen et al. (1998) found that smoking impedes collagen synthesis and recommended that patients be advised to stop smoking prior to surgery.

● *Nursing assessment* ●

(1) Cardiovascular disease: previous/present history.
(2) If wound on lower limbs, observe: skin colour
                                      warm/cold legs
                                      presence/absence pedal pulses
                                      oedema.
(3) If known Hb (normal limits 12–18 g/dl)
             pO_2 (normal limits 11–15 kPa).

2.2.4 Eating and drinking

The activity of eating is essential for health and well-being. It is also essential for wound healing. The particular nutrients that are required have been reviewed by McLaren (1993) and are summarised in Table 2.2. Many studies have considered the importance of nutrition to wound healing. Haydock and Hill (1986) found impaired wound healing in malnourished surgical patients. In a further study (1987) they found that wound healing was improved by giving intravenous nutrition to malnourished surgical patients. Delmi et al. (1990), found that malnutrition affected mortality and morbidity in elderly patients with fractured neck of femur. Other researchers have reported similar findings (Patterson et al., 1992; Tkatch et al., 1992).

Poor nutrition may be found in patients suffering from chronic wounds. It may be associated with heavy exudate where protein is being persistently lost. Mullholland et al. (1943) found that one patient with a large pressure sore lost 5.6 g of protein in wound exudate over a 24-hour period. Nylen and Wallenius (1961) found that patients with leg ulcers lost an average of 2.6 g of protein in 24 hours. Malnutrition has also been positively correlated to the development of pressure sores. Pinch-kofsky-Devin and Kaminski (1986) assessed elderly patients for nutritional status. All the patients with severe malnutrition had pressure sores. The lower the serum albumin, the more severe was the pressure sore.

Table 2.2 The nutrients required for healing.

Nutrient	Contribution
Carbohydrates	Energy for leucocyte, macrophage and fibroblast function.
Protein	Immune response, phagocytosis, angiogenesis, fibroblast proliferation, collagen synthesis, wound remodelling.
Fats	Provision of energy, formation of new cells.
Vitamins A	Collagen synthesis and cross-linking, tensile strength of wound.
B complex	Immune response, collagen cross-linking, tensile strength of wound.
C	Collagen synthesis, wound tensile strength, neutrophil function, macrophage migration, immune response.
E	Appears to reduce tissue damage from free radical formation.
Minerals Copper	Collagen synthesis, leucocyte formation.
Iron	Collagen synthesis, oxygen delivery.
Zinc	Enhances cell proliferation, increases epithelialisation, improves collagen strength.

Malnutrition is a pathological state which results from a relative or absolute deficiency or excess of one or more essential nutrients. As protein or carbohydrates are used in the largest quantities, they are usually the deficient nutrients. This is referred to as protein–energy malnutrition or PEM.

Nutritional status

In her *Notes on Nursing, What it is and What it is Not*, Florence Nightingale (1859) said

'Every careful observer of the sick will agree in this, that thousands of patients are annually starved in the midst of plenty, from want of attention to the ways which alone make it possible for them to take food'.

More than a century later this statement is still true. McWhirter and Pennington (1994) assessed the nutritional status of 500 acutely ill patients and found 40% were undernourished on admission to hospital. Gallagher-Allred *et al.* (1996) reviewed studies involving 1327 patients which showed that 40–55% were malnourished and 12% were severely malnourished.

The initial causes of malnutrition may be related to debilitating disease, especially of the gastrointestinal tract, old age, poverty or ignorance. Once admitted to hospital, other factors become relevant. An early study by Hamilton Smith (1972) found that patients are starved for up to 12 hours prior to surgery and for varying lengths of time afterwards. Chapman (1996) found little had changed in over 20 years. She found that patients fasted for periods ranging from 4–29 hours. A long period of preoperative starvation serves to compound the effects of trauma and surgery, both of which cause marked catabolism (as discussed in Section 2.2.2 on Communicating). This catabolic state usually lasts between 6 and 18 hours. Following this, the basal metabolic rate rises leading to increased energy requirements. Unless adequate protein and carbohydrate are taken in to supply these needs, further tissue breakdown occurs resulting in muscle wasting and a negative nitrogen balance. Lee (1979) suggests that the consequences of a negative nitrogen balance include poor wound healing, impaired immunocompetence and susceptibility to infection. Whilst some patients will return to a normal diet fairly quickly and so redress the balance, others will receive only intravenous fluids. A litre of dextrose 5% contains approximately 150 kilocalories ((kcal) or 'calories'). Normal saline does not contain any at all. These fluids obviously do not provide adequate calories to meet the body's requirements.

Burn patients are particularly at risk and may continue to be so for as long as four weeks (Sutherland, 1985). Trauma, burns and pain increase the metabolic rate, further diminishing the patient's nutritional status (Arturson, 1978). Zinc, in particular, is burned up in large amounts during emotional or physical stress. Table 2.3 shows the protein and calorie requirements of different patients.

Table 2.3   Daily nutritional requirements.

Type of patient	Energy (kcal)	Protein (g)
Medical patient	1500–2000	40–70
Surgical patient	2000–3500	75–125
Severe trauma or burns	3500–5000	125–300

NB These requirements will rise in the presence of sepsis or other medical complications.

It is the responsibility of nurses to see that their patients have an adequate diet. Many patients have their meal times disrupted by medical ward rounds or being away from the ward undergoing investigations. Older et al. (1980) saw food being placed beyond the reach of a patient and then removed later without the patient ever having the chance to actually eat any of it. Delmi et al. (1990), in their study of a group of elderly patients with fractured neck of femur, found that inadequate amounts of food were consumed. It should also be noted that 80% of patients in the study were malnourished on admission. Lewis et al. (1993) studied the diet of a small group of elderly patients with leg ulcers and found their intake was below the estimated average requirement for their age-group and did not meet the requirements for healing their ulcers. A similar study by Sitton-Kent and Gilchrist (1993) of elderly hospitalised patients with chronic wounds found that they did not consume adequate levels of nutrients and in some instances had inadequate quantities on their plates.

Many things can affect the appetite such as anxiety, altered meal times, cultural differences or malaise. It is obvious that a nutritional assessment of all patients should be made on admission and at regular intervals afterwards. Goodinson (1987) has highlighted those patients at risk of developing protein–energy malnutrition (see Table 2.4).

Age

The cell metabolic rate slows with advancing years. There is also an increased risk of malnutrition. Exton Smith (1971) divided the causes into primary and secondary. Primary causes included ignorance, social isolation, physical disability, mental disturbance, iatrogenic disorder and poverty. Secondary causes were impaired appetite, masticatory inefficiency, malabsorption, alcoholism, drugs and increased requirements.

Table 2.4 Conditions increasing the risk of malnutrition.

Group/condition	Possible causes/contributing factors
The elderly	Restricted resources for purchasing and storing food, poor dental status, social isolation, depression and bereavement.
Crohn's disease Ulcerative colitis	Malabsorption of nutrients, decreased intestinal transit time, diarrhoea.
Gastrointestinal surgery	Protein losses in fistula and wound exudate, increased metabolic requirements for protein/energy, period of postoperative nil by mouth.
Renal, hepatic pancreatic disease	Impose specialist nutrient requirements for protein/energy.
Arthritis	Immobility, inability to manipulate cutlery or prepare food, depression.
Cerebrovascular trauma/ disease, e.g. stroke	Sensory and motor deficits may impair perception of food, taste, smell, mastication, swallowing, weakness/paralysis unconsciousness.
Burns, trauma, injury, sepsis	Increased metabolic requirements for protein, energy and micronutrients.
Carcinoma	Taste changes, food aversions, anorexia, nausea, vomiting, diarrhoea may occur as a consequence of the disease and its treatment by chemotherapy/radiotherapy. Carcinoma of the oesophagus, pharynx and gut may constitute mechanical obstruction to intake of food.
Acute and chronic pain	Anorexia, side-effects of analgesic/medications.
Respiratory diseases associated with dyspnoea and hyperventilation	Anorexia and decreased food intake imposed by symptoms, hyperventilation increases energy requirements.
Medication	Some drugs have catabolic side-effects, e.g. corticosteroids, nausea, vomiting, diarrhoea due to side-effects of oral preparations.
Depression, grief	Anorexia, absence of interest in food.
Obesity	May be overlooked as an 'at risk' group.

From: Goodinson, S.M. (1987) *Professional Nurse*, **2** (11), 368.
By courtesy of Austen-Cornish Publishers Ltd.

Disease

Diabetes mellitus: uncontrolled glycosuria causes a weak inflammatory response and a reduction in the number of macrophages. Therefore, there is an increased risk of infection and poor healing.

Jaundice: jaundice increases the risk of abdominal dehiscence twelve-fold, particularly when associated with malignant disease (Irvin *et al.*, 1978). Taube *et al.* (1981) found that when they added bilirubin to tissue cultures of fibroblasts there were changes in cellular structure and impaired growth of the cells. However, the clinical significance of this is not certain.

Malignant disease: many patients suffering from malignant disease have a reduced nutritional status. Stubbs (1989) found that one in four cancer patients experienced alterations in taste perception which affected their appetite and eating habits.

Drugs

Several drugs affect the nutritional status of patients. Methotrexate has an anti-vitamin effect. This means that the enzyme which would normally bind a vitamin binds the drug instead. Methotrexate competes with folic acid and causes it to be excreted, thereby inhibiting DNA synthesis and cell replication (Holmes, 1986). Neomycin reduces the absorption of vitamins K and D. Para-amino-salicylic acid (PAS) and colchicine reduce the absorption of vitamin B_{12}. A number of drugs can cause a loss of appetite which may lead to a diminished nutritional status. Examples are metformin, indomethacin, morphine, digoxin and cancer drugs.

Smoking

Smoking may act as an appetite depressant. Smokers have been found to be deficient in vitamins B_1, B_6, B_{12} and C.

It should also be noted that patients not deemed to be at risk of undernutrition may fail to eat adequately. A study was undertaken by Brown (1991) of patients considered to have no special dietary requirements. She found 68% had intakes of less than 1000 kcal and large deficits of a range of vitamins and minerals. The deficit was caused by failure to eat the food provided. Adequate monitoring of patients' diets is essential.

Hunt (1997) and her colleagues have devised a nutritional assessment tool which considers various factors which can affect nutritional status. It was devised with patients with wounds in mind. Patients are assessed according to their mental condition, weight, appetite, ability to eat, gut function, medical condition including chronic wounds and age. The tool provides a score which indicates whether the patient is nutritionally at risk. Such a tool can be helpful in identifying those less obviously at risk of poor nutritional status than those discussed above.

● *Nursing assessment* ●

(1) On admission:

    (a) Identify those at special risk (Table 2.4).
    (b) Take a dietary history.
    (c) Observe for obvious signs of obesity, emaciation or muscle wasting.
    (d) Weigh patient and compare with 'usual weight'. Any weight change can be calculated with the formula

$$\frac{\text{usual weight} - \text{current weight}}{\text{current weight}} \times 100$$

    NB this measurement has no value in obesity, fluid retention or dehydration.
    If there is any indication of protein–energy malnutrition (PEM) then the following tests may be used.

(2) Anthropometric measurements: measure skin fold thickness at biceps, triceps, subscapular and suprailiac crest. The sum of these measurements should be at least 40 cm.

(3) Serum proteins: albumin (normal values 35–50 g/l) it has a half-life of 19 days and so does not change rapidly enough to be an accurate marker, but will indicate chronic PEM; transferrin (normal values 0.12–0.2 g/l) it has a half-life of 9 days and so is a more accurate measure of protein status.

(4) Nitrogen balance: measurement of protein intake and nitrogen output in urine or wound drainage. If output exceeds input then patient is in negative balance.

● *Nursing interventions* ●

Problem: Reduced nutritional status.
Goal: Patients will consume sufficient nutrients for their daily needs.

The nutritional needs of each individual vary according to their age, sex, activity and the severity of any illness. Patients who have been assessed as having a reduced nutritional status, or who fall into a high-risk category, should have their nutritional intake very carefully monitored. All patients require sufficient nutrients to support their basal metabolic rate, level of activity and metabolic response to trauma. Patients with heavily exuding wounds, such as fistulae or leg ulcers, may lose large amounts of protein without it being realised.

    The dietitian will be able to help in assessing individual needs, so that very specific goals can be set. The goal set at the beginning of this section is of necessity broad, but needs to be more clearly defined for each individual. If a patient is being cared for at home, the carer must also be involved. Many patients will eat better at home, where they can eat what they want, when they want to.

The elderly may have special problems or needs. Penfold and Crowther (1989) have provided helpful guidelines for assisting the elderly to maintain a good diet. One problem may be developing disability. The occupational therapist can give guidance on adapting cooking equipment. Another problem may be lack of education as to what constitutes a 'good' diet. An even simpler problem may be poorly fitting dentures. A new set of teeth may be all that is needed to allow an elderly person to maintain an adequate nutritional status.

For many people, the short period of starvation during surgery followed by a rapid return to an adequate diet will not be harmful and the body will quickly adapt. However, nurses need to be aware of the amount of food their patients actually eat. These days the plated meal system is widely used in hospitals and there is little monitoring of the amount that patients eat. When assisting a patient to plan appropriate menus, it is helpful to bear in mind the sources of the nutrients particularly required for wound healing (see Table 2.5).

Table 2.5 Sources of nutrients required for wound healing.

Nutrient	RDA*	Food source
Protein	42–84 g	Meat, fish, eggs, cheese, pulses, wholegrain cereals.
Carbohydrates	1600–3350 kcals	Wholemeal bread, wholegrain cereals, potatoes, (refined carbohydrates are seen as 'empty' calories).
Vitamins A	750 µg	Carrots, spinach, broccoli, apricots, melon.
B_{12}	3 mg	Meat (especially liver), dairy products, fish.
C	30 mg	Fruit and vegetables (but easily lost in cooking).
D	10 µg	Oily fish, margarine, cod liver oil.
K		Vegetables, cereals.
Minerals		
Iron	10–12 mg	Meat (especially offal), eggs, dried fruit.
Copper		Shellfish, liver, meat, bread.
Manganese		Tea, nuts, spices, whole cereals.
Zinc	12–15 mg	Oyster meat, whole cereals, cheese.

*Recommended Daily Allowance. These are the requirements in health; may need to be increased (see text).

Some critically ill patients will not have an adequate intake without artificial feeding. This may take the form of a supplement or total nutrition. It can be either by enteral or parenteral feeding. Enteral feeding is the more desirable way of providing nutrition, but if the gastrointestinal tract is not functioning, then total parenteral nutrition is necessary. Zainal (1995) discussed the issues concerning the feeding of critically ill patients and stressed the importance of starting feeds early.

● *Evaluation* ●

Evaluation may be achieved by regular weighing of the patient and by monitoring serum proteins and nitrogen output.

2.2.5 Eliminating

Uraemia inhibits fibroblast activity, but how this occurs is not yet understood (Lawrence & Payne, 1984). McDermott *et al.* (1971) also found that epithelial cell division is depressed. Patients undergoing long-term peritoneal dialysis have a high wound complication following surgery which was seen to be related to poor nutrition and a high urea (Moffat *et al.*, 1982). Barton and Barton (1981) found that a blood urea above 7 mmol/l seriously delayed both granulation and epithelialisation.

Incontinence, either urinary or faecal, causes problems of contamination in wounds in the perianal area. They are problematic to dress because of the constant soiling of the dressing.

● *Nursing assessment* ●

(1) Past or present medical history.
(2) Blood urea (normal limits 3.0–6.5 mmol/l).

2.2.6 Personal cleansing and dressing

Poor standards of personal hygiene can affect wound healing because of the increased risk of wound contamination. This may be related to socioeconomic factors (see also Maintaining a safe environment, Section 2.2.1).

● *Nursing assessment* ●

(1) Nursing history.
(2) Observation of personal habits/living accommodation.

2.2.7 Controlling body temperature

Pyrexia may be indicative of infection (see Maintaining a safe environment, Section 2.2.1). Closs (1985) found a 100% association between perioperative pyrexia and the later development of respiratory infection. However, this finding was not supported in a later study by Payman *et al.* (1989). Pyrexia is a debilitating condition which increases the metabolic rate and is often accompanied by anorexia and dehydration. It may also cause restlessness.

Hypothermia causes a shutdown of the blood supply to the periphery. The blood supply to wounds on the limbs is likely to be severely curtailed. The surface of the wound may become quite necrotic as a result.

● *Nursing assessment* ●

Monitor temperature four hourly or daily, according to the condition of the patient and to the degree of risk of infection.

2.2.8 Mobilising

People with reduced mobility may have problems with wound healing. Reduced mobility causes stasis in the peripheral circulation, especially the legs. This often results in stasis oedema and delay in the removal of waste products. Injuries to the legs are slow to heal.

Reduced mobility may also increase the risk of wound development, i.e. pressure sores. This should be taken into account when assessing patients. This topic is explored further in Chapter 5.

Drugs

Steroids and rheumatoid drugs have an anti-inflammatory effect. Steroids reduce protein synthesis, capillary budding, fibroblast proliferation and epithelialisation (Lawrence & Payne, 1984). This is probably only of significance in those patients with chronic wounds who are undergoing long-term drug therapy. Grunbine *et al.* (1998) studied 73 patients who had a steroid injection following surgery to the foot or ankle and compared the outcome with those who did not. The use of a single dose of steroids made no difference to healing rates. Studies have shown that vitamin A will counteract the ill-effects of long-term use of steriods (Salmela & Ahonen, 1984).

● *Nursing assessment* ●

(1) Nursing history – degree of mobility.
(2) Physical examination: evidence of oedema, deformity of joints/limbs.
(3) Risk assessment – see Chapter 5.

● *Nursing interventions* ●

Problem: Reduced mobility following injury/surgery/illness.
Goal: Patients will regain their previous level of mobility.

Illness from whatever cause can produce feelings of debility. Rest is necessary and a period of time may be spent in bed. As a result of injury or surgery, the patient may find it difficult to move. In most cases sufferers will regain their previous level of mobility as they start to recover. A plan of care should include simple exercises to be undertaken whilst in bed and gradual increases in activity once mobilising. A series of short-term realistic goals may be helpful to both the patient and the nurse. Advice should also be given on the levels of activity to follow after discharge from hospital.

Problem: Reduced mobility due to disability.
Goal: Patients will be able to optimise functional mobility.

Disability may occur for many reasons and has many levels of severity. Many disabilities result in reduced mobility and immobility is a potential problem. Immobility affects the cardiovascular, respiratory, gastrointestinal, urinary and musculoskeletal systems. The consequences of immobility are far reaching as shown by Figure 2.3. The patient will need to understand these potential problems and how best to avoid them. A multidisciplinary approach is the most effective way of establishing a

Immobility

Within hours:

Venous stasis due to lack of muscular massage.

Postural oedema of feet and ankles from sitting with legs down.
Stiffness of joints and muscles.

Incontinence as unable to get to toilet/commode

This may lead to:

DVT, pulmonary embolism, skin breakdown

Intractable stiffness, muscular weakness, joint contractures e.g. dropped foot

After days

Constipation;
Dehydration due to low fluid intake;
Pressure sores;
Muscular atrophy from disuse;
Chest infection because of poor ventilation
Postural hypotension because postural receptors not activated
Reduced nutritional status due to loss of appetite or poor food

This may lead to:

Faecal impaction;
Frequency of micturition with oliguria, urinary tract infection, septicaemia;
Loss of confidence;

Pneumonia;
Fainting, falls, fractures;

Deficiencies, gastric irritation

After weeks

Loss of social contact;
Deficiency syndromes, e.g. poor healing, anaemia, loss of bone density, weight loss;
Loss of ability to care for self

This may lead to:

Depression, purposelessness; confusion; heart failure

Contributes to hypothermia if person falls

Eventually: Difficulty in rehabilitating
Further immobility
Death

Fig. 2.3 The consequences of immobility.

suitable plan of care for those with major disability. This will ensure that all team members reinforce all aspects of the plan of care. Again, short-term goals are the most effective as they provide a sense of achievement as each goal is reached.

Disability does not just gradually disappear. Patients must be prepared for the return to the community. Adaptations to the home may be required. Family or any significant others must be involved in planning and learning to manage any aspects of care that may be needed. Involvement of community staff must also be established. Appropriate long-term strategies can be established which optimise the patient's abilities whilst preventing potential problems.

● *Evaluation* ●

Continuous evaluation of progress towards goals will enable the constant adaptation of goals to realistic levels.

2.2.9 Expressing sexuality

Body image is the mental picture that people have of themselves. Sexuality is an integral part of the image. Body image is also closely associated with self-esteem. Shipes (1987) suggests that self-esteem can be defined as the sum total of all we believe about ourselves. All patients with wounds have an altered body image. This can have a profound effect on self-esteem and motivation. Obvious types of wounds which can have these effects are those resulting in disfigurement such as burns, head and neck surgery, mastectomy, amputation and ostomies. Many patients will also be suffering from anxiety about their prognosis. The resultant stress can be so overwhelming that patients may be unable to take in information, to share their feelings or to commence rehabilitation. This has physiological effects which delay wound healing (see also Communicating, Section 2.2.2, and Psychological care, Section 2.3).

● *Nursing assessment* ●

An assessment has been suggested by Shipes (1987). It was developed for ostomy patients, but could also be used for other patients.

- Value attached to altered/missing part (could be cultural values).
- Meaning of altered body to patient.
- Support system: family, friends?
- Current activities and plans for the future.
- Evidence of negative self-esteem?
  - refuses to touch or look at wound.
  - refuses to discuss wound.
  - verbalises feelings of worthlessness.
  - refuses to participate in care.
  - withdraws from social contacts.
  - avoids intimate relationships.
  - poor grooming.

● *Nursing interventions* ●

Problem: Loss of self-esteem related to altered body image.
Goal: Patients acknowledge change in body image and expresses their feelings about this change.

In the early stages, following the circumstances which led to an altered body image, some patients appear to be quite euphoric. This is due to simple relief at having survived. After a while the patient's attitude is likely to change. Common problems that can occur include:

- a sense of loss, similar to bereavement
- anxiety related to diagnosis, especially if it is cancer
- loss of sexual function which may be related to type of surgery or trauma or to either of the previous problems
- a withdrawal from social relationships with family or significant others, possibly due to a malodorous wound or any of the previous problems.

The role of the nurse is to assist the patient to develop a re-integrated body image (Burgess, 1994). This may be achieved in a variety of ways. Perhaps the most important is to accept the patient as he is, at whatever stage he has reached. Allowing a patient to express his feelings and providing him with matter-of-fact information, such as an honest appraisal of the progress of his wound, is beneficial. It is also essential to include family and/or significant others in the patient's care and in any education programme. Good management of the wound should prevent odour or leakage which helps to boost confidence. Burgess also suggests that if patients are having difficulty coping it may be necessary to emphasise the importance of the surgery for the health of the individual and the fact that it does not change them as a person.

As already discussed under Communicating (Section 2.2.2), preoperative information and counselling are most important. Kelly (1989) studied 67 patients who had undergone head and neck surgery. Generally, they said they were more anxious before surgery than after. Some 42% of men and 21% of women would have liked more information. Another study by Elspie *et al.* (1989) found that 41% of patients suffered psychological stress following major surgery for intraoral cancer.

In many areas, specialist nurses are employed to give help and support to patients, such as stoma nurses or breast care nurses. They can build up a relationship with their patients which give the patients the confidence to express their feelings freely. In other circumstances, it may be a nurse who has a good relationship with a patient who is able to provide this service.

● *Evaluation* ●

Regular evaluation of progress is important for patients with an altered body image. Learning to cope with the new image may take time, and strategies may have to be altered along the way. This may be particularly true for those undergoing a series of plastic surgery operations. They may have to cope with a constantly changing body image.

2.2.10 Sleeping

In recent years there has been considerable research on sleep and its effects. Sleep deprivation causes people to become increasingly irritable and irrational (Carter, 1985). They may complain of lassitude and loss of feelings of well-being. The sleep–activity cycle is part of the circadian rhythms. During wakefulness the body is in a state of catabolism. Hormones such as catecholamine and cortisol are released.

They encourage tissue degradation to provide energy for activity, in particular, protein degradation occurs in muscle. Growth hormone is secreted from the anterior pituitary during sleep. Lee and Stotts (1990) have reviewed the role of growth hormone in wound healing. It stimulates protein synthesis and the proliferation of a variety of cells including fibroblasts and endothelial cells.

There is much evidence that sleep patterns are disturbed in hospital. Hill (1989) suggested that ward routines, such as early morning waking, prevent the patient getting adequate sleep. Also, many patients are disturbed during the night. Walker (1972) found that cardiotomy patients were disturbed approximately 14 times an hour in the immediate postoperative period. Woods (1972) observed a similar group of patients and noted that they were disturbed as many as 56 times during the first postoperative night. Morgan and White (1983) found that intensive care nurses were aware of the importance of sleep, but failed to recognise when they were disturbing their patients unnecessarily.

Other factors may also disturb sleep such as anxiety, pain, being unable to sleep in an accustomed position, uncomfortable beds, noise and a high ambient temperature (Closs, 1990). A further study by Closs (1991) considered in greater detail the extent to which pain disturbed sleep at night. Total night-time sleep was found to be reduced by a mean of one hour compared with normal patterns. Nearly 75% reported that pain had prevented sleep. A mean of 3.3 awakenings during the night was found. Despite the fact that about 50% of patients said that their pain was worse at night, they received less analgesia during this time.

● *Nursing assessment* ●

(1) Compare 'normal' with present patterns of sleep.
(2) Assess the ward environment – is it conducive to sleeping?
(3) Consider ward routines: do they allow the patient to follow any aspect of usual routines, or are they too rigid?

● *Nursing interventions* ●

Problem: Disruption of normal sleeping patterns.
Goal: Patients are able to sleep a number of hours at night and feel well rested.

Hospitals are not restful places. Many patients joke about going home for a rest. Noise is a major factor which disturbs patients, especially irritating noises. Florence Nightingale (1859) discussed the importance of sleep to the sick. She described some of the noises that disturbed patients. They included rattling keys, creaking shoes and stays (corsets) and the rustle of clothes. Whilst at first glance this may appear quite outmoded, there is still truth in this today. Stead (1985) asked patients what disturbed them at night and found that the major problem was noise, in particular, rattling keys and squeaking shoes. Attention to noise reduction at night is an important aspect of nursing care.

McMahon (1990) suggested four types of sleeplessness:

- difficulty getting to sleep
- waking regularly during the night

- waking early in the morning
- sleeping for the normal length of time, but not waking refreshed.

Various strategies can be employed to help patients resolve their specific problems. The provision of a milky drink can be beneficial, especially if the patient normally has one at bedtime. Some people may become hungry after having supper between 5pm and 6pm. They may ask their visitors to bring them in a snack. Although there is no evidence that food can induce sleep, it is difficult to sleep when hungry. Most people have specific routines that they follow each night. As much as possible this same routine should be followed in hospital. It can introduce a feeling of normality into a strange situation.

Some people find their sleep disrupted because of pain. This may be acute pain following trauma or surgery or a more chronic pain relating to a long-standing illness or condition. Adequate pain control is essential. Pain is a resolvable problem (see also Communicating, Section 2.2.2). The position of patients may affect their comfort, it is helpful to ensure that patients are comfortable, with a bell to hand.

During the night, many fears that are suppressed during the day come to the surface. Sleep may be disturbed because of a particular anxiety. Night time is a quieter time on the ward. It may provide an opportunity for the nurse to sit and listen to patients and allow them to express their fears and anxieties. Once this has happened, patients may be able to return to their normal sleep patterns.

Hospital routines can disrupt normal sleep patterns. The lights of a ward may go off late, around 11pm and come on again at 6am (Stead, 1985). Patients are woken for their drugs and a drink. It seems not unreasonable for more flexibility to be introduced with a reduction of the 6am drug round to the minimum and an arrangement not to wake those who would prefer to sleep later. Haddock (1994) found some patients benefited from using earplugs, however, they are not suitable for everyone.

It should be possible, with careful planning, to provide an environment which is conducive to sleep, and a comfortable patient who is able to benefit from it.

● *Evaluation* ●

Patient questionnaires are a useful way of establishing the success or otherwise of the above plan.

2.2.11 Dying

When caring for terminally ill patients with wounds, there are two factors to consider. Firstly, there may not be adequate time left to the patient for a large wound to heal. Secondly, the disease process may adversely affect the healing process. It is important for these patients that appropriate goals are set for their care. These goals should consider the patients' wishes rather than what the nurse thinks they should be. Patient comfort should be of primary consideration. If the wound cannot be healed, then aggressive treatment should be abandoned and dressings which reduce frequency of dressing change utilised.

● *Nursing assessment* ●

This is not always an easy assessment and other disciplines should be involved.

(1) Identify the problems which distress the patient, e.g. pain at dressing change, heavy exudate, odour.

2.2.12 Medical/other intervention

Cancer chemotherapy

These drugs are used to destroy cancer cells throughout the body, both the primary growth and any metastases. They are most effective on rapidly dividing cells. However, they are unable to differentiate between normal and abnormal cells. The majority of drugs work by destroying DNA, or interfering with protein synthesis or cell division. This directly affects fibroblast synthesis and collagen production. Falcone and Nappi (1984) reviewed the range of drugs available and their effect on surgical wounds. They concluded that chemotherapeutic drugs should not be given perioperatively, but after seven to ten days, when the healing process has become established. A more recent study (Robinson *et al.*, 1990) of the effects of cisplatin on wound-bursting strength supported this view. Administration of the drug preoperatively or one day postoperatively had a detrimental effect which was not seen if cisplatin was given one week postoperatively.

It should also be remembered that many cancer drugs affect nutritional status by causing nausea and vomiting (see Eating and drinking, Section 2.2.4).

Radiotherapy

Radiation effectively destroys cancer cells as they are more radiosensitive than normal cells. A dosage high enough to kill cancer cells does not affect the surrounding cells. However, if the dosage has to be increased there is increased risk of normal tissue necrosing. Luce (1984) describes this as a complication and outlines the relationship between cure and complication. He concludes that, whilst a relatively low cure rate of 42–50% would entail a low incidence of complication, a complication rate of 50% would have to be accepted in order to obtain a cure rate of 80%.

Hillmann *et al.* (1997) found preoperative irradiation was an influencing factor in postoperative complications for patients with Ewing's sarcoma. The potential for complication may last for some time. Sassler *et al.* (1995) found major wound complications in patients undergoing head and neck surgery following an initial regime of chemotherapy and irradiation. They found a 77% incidence of complications in patients undergoing surgery within one year of the regime compared with a 20% incidence after one year.

Radiation may affect the healing of an existing wound or it may cause changes to the skin so that any later wound will heal slowly. The skin may show signs of damage from the radiation during treatment. This is known as a radiation reaction and will be discussed in Chapter 6.

Levenson *et al.* (1984) investigated the use of vitamin A supplements to counteract the effects of radiation on wound healing. In the animal model they found that giving vitamin A supplements was effective. Good results were obtained if the supplementation was started prior to radiotherapy or up to two days after treatment.

● *Nursing assessment* ●

(1) Patient history will indicate use of chemotherapy or radiotherapy.
(2) History of nausea or vomiting or alteration in eating habits.
(3) Nutritional assessment (see Eating and drinking, Section 2.2.4).

2.3 PSYCHOLOGICAL CARE

Nurses have always excelled at the physical care of patients. It is only recently that the emotional needs of patients have been considered. Many situations may cause psychological distress. This may be described as stress. The physiological effects of stress and its effect on wound healing have already been described in the section on Communicating (2.2.2). Factors causing psychological distress may be defined as stressors. Those which may be particularly associated with wounded patients will be discussed in this section. It should be noted that other factors not addressed here may also act as stressors.

Fear

Fear is a common human experience which may be transitory or longer lasting. Illness may release many fears – fear of hospitalisation, fear of illness, fear of a life-threatening condition, fear of loss of affection of loved ones, fear of the mutilation of surgery. Such fear creates great stress within the sufferer. This may be made worse by the healthcare team failing to recognise when patients are experiencing fear and so not allowing them to express their feelings.

Grief

Grief is a normal process which allows adaptation to some major loss in a person's life. The wounded patient may have to come to terms with skin damage from burns, the loss of a limb or breast, or other types of mutilating surgery (see also Expressing sexuality, Section 2.2.9). Kubler-Ross (1969) described various stages in the grief process. She related them to dying, but they can be applied to all types of grief. The stages are: denial, isolation, anger, bargaining, depression and acceptance (see Table 2.6). Each person will progress through some or all of these stages at a different rate and not necessarily in the same sequence. By listening to the patient and accepting without judgement, the nurse can assist in this process and thus reduce the amount of stress suffered. This may be particularly difficult during the stage of anger as the aggression expressed by the patient is often directed at the main caregivers. Understanding of the cause of the aggression will help the nurse deal with this stage of grief.

Table 2.6 The grief process.

Denial: The patient denies the situation by refusing to discuss it or walking away. This stage can be prolonged by others also denying the problem for the patient.

Isolation: The patient may withdraw within him/herself to start to cope with the situation. He/she may experience feelings of intense loneliness.

Anger: The patient may become very aggressive or critical as he feels very angry that he has been 'chosen' to suffer in this way.

Bargaining: At this stage the patient may try to delay the problem by promising good behaviour.

Depression: Once the patient can no longer deny his problem/illness the feelings of rage and disbelief are gradually replaced by a sense of loss associated with depression. This seems to be a beneficial and constructive emotion.

Acceptance: This is a sense of completion or preparedness for what has or will happen.

Based on Kubler-Ross, E. (1969).

Powerlessness

Taylor and Cress (1987) describe powerlessness as the 'perception of loss of control over what happens to oneself and one's environment'. This is a feeling experienced by many hospital patients as they are placed in the subservient 'patient role'. Even simple decisions such as when to eat or go to bed are taken away from the individual. There is pressure to conform and be a 'good' patient. Stockwell (1972) describes very graphically the fate of the unpopular patient who did not conform to the role the nurses desired from him. A 'good' patient will submit without question to treatment and will not ask too many questions. Although it is to be hoped that nursing has moved forward since 1972, many patients are still aware of their loss of status once they are in hospital. Some may feel depressed because of their feelings of learned helplessness. Others may feel quite euphoric to have survived, which may also be misinterpreted as a lack of compliance.

In a society where independence is prized, dependence on others may produce feelings of anger and frustration. Many patients remark that they feel a nuisance because they cannot care for themselves. It may also reduce their feelings of self-worth. An example might be cited of an elderly man with bilateral amputations of his legs. He felt that he had no control of his life and was nothing but a trouble to everyone. Simply being asked to take part in a small research project and then realising his contribution had been very valuable, greatly raised his self-esteem.

● *Nursing assessment* ●

Although the precise problem may vary, the assessment is the same.

(1) Observe body language: does the patient avoid eye contact, look relaxed, tense, fidgety, withdrawn, hypoactive, hyperactive?

Conversation: does the patient talk excessively, not talk to any-one, ask questions, non-questioning?

Do any of these terms describe the patient?

- angry
- aggressive
- demanding
- anxious
- critical
- depressed
- disorientated
- confused
- confident
- distrustful
- fearful
- passive
- euphoric

Katona and Katona (1997) proposed that a slightly different approach is required for assessing older people. They recommended the use of four simple questions. Are you basically satisfied with your life? Do you feel that your life is empty? Are you afraid that something bad is going to happen to you? Do you feel happy most of the time? The patient would score a point for replying no to the first and last question and for replying yes to the middle two. Anyone with a score of two or more is probably depressed.

● *Nursing interventions* ●

Although nurse training is providing improved knowledge of psychological care, it may be appropriate for the patient to have further help from others: a clinical psychologist, a psychiatric nurse, a chaplain or a trained counsellor.

Problem: Fear due to separation from loved ones or related to unfamiliarity.
Goal: Patients identify the source(s) of their fear and are able to describe their feelings.

Once the nurse has been able to recognise that the patient is very frightened, then strategies can be developed to allow the patient the opportunity to express the specific fears. Time may have to be allowed for 'casual' conversation, especially if the patient has few visitors. Assigning the same nurses to care for the patient can build up confidence. Involving the patient and, possibly, the family in all aspects of planning may be helpful. Patients with any sort of sensory loss will need orientation to the new surroundings.

Problem: Grieving related to loss of or disfigurement to a body part.
Goal: Patients will allow themselves to experience the grieving process.

A variety of strategies can be adopted to help the patient move through the grief process. Setting aside time to allow the patient to talk is very important. However, it may be constructive to set time constraints as it can be exhausting for both the patient and the nurse. Patients may prefer to know that they have the undivided attention of a nurse for a set period of time each day, rather than an indeterminate amount of time occasionally. For some individuals, it may be appropriate for others to assist the patient in recognising and talking through their grief. In those situations, the nurse should be there to support and encourage.

Problem: Powerlessness related to feelings of loss of control of the environment.

Goal: Patients will express feelings of having a sense of control and will participate in the planning of care.

Many healthcare workers fail to recognise the degree to which the 'system' takes charge of individuals once they pass through the doors of a hospital. Although in an emergency situation there may be some alteration of priorities, every patient is entitled to be treated with respect. Nurses can play an important role in assisting their patients to remain in control of as many areas of their lives as possible. Patient education not only promotes compliance, but allows the patient to participate in care, thus having a degree of control. Discussing with patients the times particular treatment should be given and involving them in planning care will reduce feelings of powerlessness.

● *Evaluation* ●

Evaluation of psychological care is not easy. Some indication can be obtained by repeating the assessment and by talking to the patient.

2.4 SPIRITUAL CARE

Spirituality is a concept with which many nurses are uncomfortable (Allen, 1991). Spirituality should not just be put into the framework of religion. Everyone, whether believing in a God or not, has spiritual needs. Spirituality can be defined as that within us that responds to the infinite realities of life. Peck (1987) described four sequential stages of spiritual development – chaotic, formal, sceptic and mystic. Whilst some may never progress beyond the first stage, others may do so and then regress during times of emotional stress.

Spiritual needs were identified by Fish and Shelley (1985) as the need for meaning and purpose, the need for love and relatedness and the need for forgiveness. Highfield and Cason (1983) also added the need for hope and creativity. Work by Simsen (1986) gave further insight into each person's need for meaning and purpose in life. A patient will seek to understand why he is suffering in a particular way. Until the patient has found meaning to his disease he cannot cope with what will happen next. Once he has, he can move on to the next stage. Simsen describes it as a continuous pattern – the search for meaning and purpose in life followed by experiencing the meaning which leads to anticipating new meaning. Simsen argues that this can be achieved by the promotion of hope and trust, mediated by good relationships.

If the spiritual needs of individuals are not met, or they experience a catastrophic event in their lives, the result is spiritual pain or distress. Morrison (1992) discussed spiritual pain and suggested it was the result of the shattering of a person's view of life resulting in a loss of meaning. Spiritual distress is recognised by the North American Nursing Diagnosis Association as a nursing diagnosis. (Within the UK, the term 'actual' or 'potential problem' is generally used instead of nursing diagnosis.) Spiritual distress is defined by Kim *et al.* (1987) as 'a disruption in the life principle that pervades a person's entire being and that integrates and transcends one's biological nature'. The effect of this is not only on the spirit or the emotions, but also physical. Spiritual distress is a stressor which can affect healing. (See also Communicating (Section 2.2.2) and Psychological care (Section 2.3).)

Spiritual distress can show in a variety of ways. The following are examples of loss of meaning and purpose in life, hopelessness and a need for forgiveness:

- A long-term paraplegic lady found that she was no longer 'in charge' of her large family because of a lengthy stay in hospital. Her purpose and meaning in life had been lost. She became withdrawn and irritable and lost her appetite.

- A patient suffering from multiple sclerosis had become much more disabled and developed pressure sores. She lost all hope in her circumstances and became extremely withdrawn, refusing to be with others and avoiding all eye contact.

- An elderly man, aware that his disease was in its terminal stages became extremely distressed, but would not discuss the reason for this. His son explained that he had not spoken to his brother for 20 years. The man wanted to be forgiven by his brother but did not know how to ask him.

In the context of spiritual distress, acceptance also has significance. A patient may need reassurance that others, particularly family and friends, will accept him/her in the new role as a patient, especially if having to come to terms with a disfiguring wound.

● *Nursing assessment* ●

(1) The patient may:

- express concern about the meaning of life and death
- show anger towards God/others
- question the meaning of suffering/illness/forms of treatment
- question the value of his own existence and that of others
- describe inner conflicts about beliefs
- appear withdrawn and lacking in response
- show loss of appetite
- sleep a great deal/not sleep (afraid of not waking)
- show less interest in treatment and care

(2) The patient may make comments such as:

- 'Why is this happening to me?'
- 'I've never done anyone any harm'
- 'I must have been very wicked to have to suffer all this'
- 'There's always someone worse off than yourself'
- 'These things are meant to try us'.

● *Nursing interventions* ●

Problem: Spiritual distress related to separation from religious or cultural ties or from a challenged belief or value system.

Goal: Patients will be able to identify the cause of spiritual distress and specify the assistance required to alleviate it.

Many nurses feel uncomfortable with this type of problem and may seek to avoid or ignore it (Stepnick & Perry, 1992). They may perceive that the only necessary nursing intervention is to arrange for the patient to attend a service in the chapel. Although many patients find great comfort from this, spiritual care should be seen in much wider terms. The chaplaincy team can give much support to both the patients and staff by listening, comforting and counselling when necessary. However, nurses need to have some understanding of the aspects of spiritual care.

There can be no standardised nursing care as there is with postoperative physical care. In this situation, individual patients must be cared for in the light of their own needs. Even without strong spiritual beliefs, a nurse can provide spiritual care. Carson (1989) suggests that the most effective way of giving spiritual care is the nurse's offering of self. She goes on to describe this as 'being present so as to touch another's spirit'. Fish and Shelly (1985) list five requirements necessary to be able to achieve this: listening, empathy, vulnerability, humility and commitment.

Listening: This is active listening, giving the patient full attention and noting all the non-verbal as well as verbal cues.

Empathy: This allows the nurse to share the feelings of the patient without losing objectivity. This is essential to enable the patient to consider alternatives.

Vulnerability: As the nurse enters into and shares the patient's feelings, she becomes vulnerable. This may be painful, but can also be rewarding.

Humility: This is not easy, few people want to admit that they do not have the answers in their particular field. A sense of humility will enable nurses to see that they can learn from their patients. Humility also allows nurses to accept themselves and their patients in all their human frailty.

Commitment: Being with a patient through all the difficult times, sharing the pain as well as the joys, involves considerable commitment.

● *Evaluation* ●

Just as spiritual assessment is very difficult, so too is evaluation of the outcomes of care. Narayanasamy (1996) suggests that spiritual integrity is one outcome which may be demonstrated as relief from spiritual pain or by restoration of the life principle. Spiritual integrity may also be shown by the development of meaningful, purposeful behaviour or a reality-based tranquillity (O'Brien, 1982).

REFERENCES

Allen, C. (1991) The inner light. *Nursing Standard*, **5** (20), 52–53.

Altemeier, W.A., Burke, J.F., Pruitt, B.A., Sandusky, W.R. (1984) *Manual on Control of Infection in Surgical Patients*. J.B. Lippincott, Philadelphia.

Arturson, M.G.S. (1978) Metabolic changes following thermal injury. *World Journal of Surgery*, **2**, 203–213.

Ayliffe, G.A., Collins, B.J., Taylor, L.J. (1982) *Hospital-Acquired Infection, Principles and Prevention*. P.S.G. Wright, Bristol.

Barton, A., Barton, M. (1981) *The Management and Prevention of Pressure Sores*. Faber and Faber, London.

Beddows, J. (1997) Alleviating pre-operative anxieties in patients: a study. *Nursing Standard*, **11** (37), 35–38.

Bibby, B.A., Collins, B.J., Ayliffe, G.A.J. (1986) A mathematical model for assessing the risk of post-operative wound infection. *Journal of Hospital Infection*, **8**, 31–39.

Birkmeyer, N.J., Charlesworth, D.C., Hernandez, F., Leavitt, B.J., Marrin, C.A., Morton, J.R., *et al.* (1998) Obesity and risk of adverse outcomes associated with coronary artery bypass surgery. Northern New England Cardiovascular Disease Study Group. *Circulation*, **97** (17), 1689–1694.

Blaylock, J. (1968) Psychological and cultural influences on the reaction to pain. *Nursing Forum*, **7**, 271–272.

Boore, J. (1978) *Prescription for Recovery*. RCN Publications, London.

Borger, M.A., Rao, V., Weisel, R.D., Ivanov, J., Cohen, G., Scully, H.E., David, T.E. (1998) Deep sternal wound infection: risk factors and outcomes. *Annals of Thoracic Surgery*, **65** (4), 1050–1056.

Bowell, B. (1992) Protecting the patient at risk. *Nursing Times*, **88** (3), 32–35.

Brown, K. (1991) Improving intakes. *Nursing Times*, **87** (20), 64–68.

Burgess, L. (1994) Facing the reality of head and neck cancer. *Nursing Standard*, **8** (32), 30–34.

Carr, E. (1997) Overcoming barriers to effective pain control. *Professional Nurse*, **12** (6), 412–416.

Carr, E., Thomas, V.J. (1997) Anticipating and experiencing post-operative pain: the patients' perspective. *Journal of Clinical Nursing*, **6**, 191–201.

Carson, V.B. (1989) *Spiritual Dimensions in Nursing Practice*, W.B. Saunders Company, Philadelphia.

Carter, D. (1985) In need of a good night's sleep. *Nursing Times*, **81** (46), 24–26.

Chan, A.W., Macfarlane, I.A., Bowsher, D. (1990) Chronic pain in patients with diabetes mellitus: comparison with a non-diabetic population. *Pain Clinic*, **3** (3), 147–159.

Chapman, A. (1996) Current theory and practice: a study of pre-operative fasting. *Nursing Standard*, **10** (18), 33–36.

Chmell, M.J., Schwartz, H.S. (1996) Analysis of variables affecting wound healing after musculoskeletal sarcoma resections. *Journal of Surgical Oncology*, **61**, 185–189.

Closs, S.J. (1985) Body composition and post-operative hypothermia. Unpublished MPhil thesis, Nottingham University.

Closs, S.J. (1990) Influences on patients' sleep on surgical wards. *Surgical Nurse*, **3** (2), 12–14.

Closs, S.J. (1991) Postoperative pain at night. *Nursing Times*, **87** (18), 40.

Closs, S.J. (1992) Patients' night time pain, analgesic provision and sleep after surgery. *International Journal of Nursing Studies*, **29** (4), 381–392.

Cook, T.D. (1984) Major research analysis provides proof patient education does make a difference. *Promoting Health*, **5** (9), 4–5.

Cruse, P.J.E., Foord, R. (1973) A five-year prospective study of 23,649 surgical wounds. *Archives of Surgery*, **107**, 206–217.

Cruse, P.J.E., Foord, R. (1980) The epidemiology of wound infection. *Surgical Clinics of North America*, **60** (1), 27–40.

Dale, F. (1993) Post-operative pain in the elective surgical patient. *British Journal of Nursing*, **2** (17), 842–849.

Delmi, M., Rapin, C.H., Bengoa, J.M. (1990) Dietary supplementation in elderly patients with fractured neck of femur. *Lancet*, **235**, 1013–1016.

Department of Health (1990) *Health Service Management – Patient Consent to Examination and Treatment*. Department of Health, NHS Management Executive, London.

Dossey, B. (1991) Awakening the inner healer. *American Journal of Nursing*, **Aug.**, 31–34.

Elspie, C.A., Freedlander, E., Campsie, L.M. *et al.* (1989) Psychological distress at follow-up after major surgery for intraoral cancer. *Journal of Psychosomatic Research*, **33** (4), 441–448.

Emmerson, A.M., Enstone, J.E., Griffin, M., Kelsey, M.C., Smyth, E.T.M. (1996) The second national prevalence survey of infection in hospitals – overview of the results. *Journal of Hospital Infection*, **32**, 175–190.

Exton-Smith, A.N. (1971) Nutrition of the elderly. *British Journal of Hospital Medicine*, **5**, 639–645.

Fagerhaugh, S.Y., Strauss, A. (1977) *Politics of Pain Management: Staff-Patient Interaction*. Addison-Wesley, London.

Falcone, R.E., Nappi, J.F. (1984) Chemotherapy and wound healing. *Surgical Clinics of North America*, **64** (4), 779–794.

Fernie, Q.R., Dornan, J. (1976) The problem of clinical trials with new systems for preventing or healing decubiti, in (eds) Kenedi, R.M., Dowden, J.M., Scales, J.T., *Bedsore Biomechanics*. Macmillan Press, London.

Field, L. (1996) Are nurses still underestimating patients' pain post-operatively? *British Journal of Nursing*, **5** (13), 778–784.

Fish, S., Shelley, J.A. (1985) *Spiritual Care: the nurse's role*. InterVarsity Press, Downers Grove, IL.

Frankenhaeuser, M. (1967) Some aspects of research in physiological psychology, in (ed) Levi, L., *Emotional Stress, Physiological and Psychological Reactions – Medical, Industrial and Military Implications*. Karger, Basel.

Gallagher-Allred, C.R., Voss, A.C., Finn, S.C., McCamish, M.A. (1996) Malnutrition and clinical outcomes: a case for medical nutrition therapy. *Journal of American Dietetic Association*, **96** (4), 361–366.

Goodinson, S.M. (1987) Assessment of nutritional status. *Professional Nurse*, **2** (11), 367–369.

Gould, D. (1992) Hygienic hand decontamination. *Nursing Standard*, **6** (32), 33–36.

Grunbine, N., Dobrowolski, C., Bernstein, A. (1998) Retrospective evaluation of post-operative steroid injections on wound healing. *Journal of Foot & Ankle Surgery*, **37** (2), 135–144.

Haddock, J. (1994) Reducing the effects of noise in hospital. *Nursing Standard*, **8** (43), 25–28.

Hamilton Smith, A. (1972) *Nil by Mouth*. RCN Publications, London.

Harmer, M., Davies, K.A. (1998) The effect of education, assessment and a standardised prescription for post-operative pain management. The value of clinical audit in the establishment of acute pain services. *Anaesthesia*, **53** (5), 424–430.

Haydock, D.A., Hill, G.L. (1986) Impaired wound healing in surgical patients with varying degrees of malnutrition. *Journal of Enteral and Parenteral Nutrition*, **10** (6), 550–554.

Haydock, D.A., Hill, G.L. (1987) Improved wound healing response in surgical patients receiving intravenous nutrition. *British Journal of Surgery*, **74**, 320–323.

Hayward, J. (1975) *Information – a Prescription against Pain*. RCN Publications, London.

He, G.W., Ryan, W.H., Acuff, T.E., Bowman, R.T., Douthit, M.B., Yang, C.Q., Mack, M.J. (1994) Risk factors for operative mortality and sternal wound infection in bilateral internal mammary artery grafting. *Journal of Thoracic & Cardiovascular Surgery*, **107** (1), 196–202.

Heidt, P. (1981) Effect of therapeutic touch on anxiety level of hospitalised patients. *Nursing Research*, **30** (1), 32–37.

Hicks, F., Simpson, K.H., Tosh, G.C. (1994) Management of spinal infusions in palliative care. *Palliative Medicine*, **8** (4), 325–332.

Highfield, M.F., Cason, C. (1983) Spiritual needs of patients: are they recognised? *Cancer Nursing*, **6**, 187–192.

Hill, J. (1989) A good night's sleep. *Senior Nurse*, **9** (5), 17–19.

Hillmann, A., Ozaki, T., Rube, C., Hoffman, C., Schuck, A., Blasius, *et al.* (1997) Surgical complications after pre-operative irradiation of Ewing's sarcoma. *Journal of Cancer Research and Clinical Oncology*, **123** (1), 57–62.

Hitchcock, L.S., Ferrell, B.R., McCaffery, M. (1994) The experience of chronic non-malignant pain. *Journal of Pain and Symptom Management*, **9** (5), 312–318.

Holden-Lund, C. (1988) Effects of relaxation with guided imagery on surgical stress and wound healing. *Research Nursing Health*, **11** (4), 235–244.

Holmes, S. (1986) Nutritional needs of medical patients. *Nursing Times*, **82** (16), 34–36.

Holzman, A.D., Turk, D.C. (1986) *Pain Management*. Pergamon Press, Oxford.

Horton R. (1993) Introducing high quality infection control in a hospital setting. *British Journal of Nursing*, **2** (15), 746–754.

Hunt, A. (1997) Assessment and planning for older people. *Nursing Times*, **93** (21), 74–78.

Irvin, T.T., Vassilakis, J.S., Chattopadhyay, D.K., Greaney, M.G. (1978) Abdominal healing in jaundiced patients. *British Journal of Surgery*, **65**, 521–522.

Janis, I.L. (1958) *Psychological Stress*. Wiley, New York.

Jorgensen, L.N., Kallehave, F., Christensen, E., Siana, J.E., Gottrup, F. (1998) Less collagen production in smokers. *Surgery*, **123** (4), 450–455.

Katona, C.L., Katona, P.M. (1997) Geriatric depression scale can be used in older people in primary care. *British Medical Journal*, **315** (7117), 1236.

Kelly, R. (1989) *A study of patients who have had surgery in the head and neck region.* Paper given at the RCN Research Scotland Symposium, Nov.

Kiecolt-Glaser, J.K., Marucha, P.T., Malarkey, W.B., Mercado, A.M., Glaser, R. (1995) Slowing of wound healing by psychological stress. *Lancet*, **346** (8984), 1194–1196.

Kim, M.J., McFarland, G.K., McLane, A.M. (1987) *Pocket Guide to Nursing Diagnoses*, 2nd edn. C.V. Mosby, St Louis.

Kinney, J.M. (1977) The metabolic response to injury, in (eds) Richards, J.R., Kinney, J.M., *Nutritional Aspects of the Critically Ill*. Churchill-Livingstone, Edinburgh.

Knighton, D.R., Silver, I.A., Hunt, T.K. (1981) Regulation of wound healing angiogenesis – effect of oxygen gradients and inspired oxygen concentration. *Surgery*, **90**, 262–270.

Koshy, K.T. (1989) I only have ears for you. *Nursing Times*, **85** (30), 26–29.

Kubler-Ross, E. (1969) *On Death and Dying*. Macmillan, London.

Larson, E., Kretzer, E.K. (1995) Compliance with handwashing and barrier precautions. *Journal of Hospital Infection*, **30** Suppl., 88–106.

Lawrence, J.C., Payne, H.J. (1984) *Wound Healing*. The Update Group, London.

Lazarus, R.S., Averill, J.R. (1972) Emotion and cognition with special reference to anxiety, in (ed) Spielberger, C.D., *Anxiety: Current Trends in Theory and Research*. Academic Press, New York.

Lee, H.A. (1979) Why enteral nutrition? *Research and Clinical Forums*, **1**, 15–24.

Lee, K.A., Stotts, N.A. (1990) Support of the growth hormone–somatomedin system to facilitate wound healing. *Heart Lung*, **19** (2), 157–163.

Levenson, S.M., Gruber, C.A., Rettura, G., Gruber, D.K., Demetriou, A.A., Seifter, E. (1984) Supplemental Vitamin A prevents acute radiation-induced deficit in wound healing. *Annals of Surgery*, **200**, 494–512.

Lewis, B.K., Hitchings, H., Bale, S., Harding, K.G. (1993) Nutritional status of elderly patients with venous ulceration of the leg – report of a pilot study. *Journal of Human Nutrition & Dietetics*, **6**, 509–515.

Luce, E.A. (1984) The irradiated wound. *Surgical Clinics of North America*, **64** (4), 821–829.

McDermot, F.T., Nauman, J., De Boer, W.G. (1971) Epithelial cell division in acute renal failure. A radio-autographic study in the oesophagus of the mouse. *British Journal of Surgery*, **58**, 52–55.

McLaren, S. (1993) Nutritional factors in wound healing. *Wound Management*, **3** (1), 8–10.

McMahon, R. (1990) Sleep therapies. *Surgical Nursing*, **3** (5), 17–20.

McPhee, I.B., Williams, R.P., Swanson, C.E. (1998) Factors influencing wound healing after surgery for metastatic disease of the spine. *Spine*, **23** (6), 726–732.

McWhirter, J.P., Pennington, C.R. (1994) Incidence and recognition of malnutrition in hospital. *British Medical Journal*, **308** (6934), 945–948.

Marshall, M. (1991) Stress management in dermatology patients. *Nursing Standard*, **5** (24), 29–31.

Martens, M.G., Kolrud, B.L., Faro, S., Maccato, M., Hammill, H. (1995) Development of wound infection or separation after caesarian delivery. Prospective evaluation of 2431 cases. *Journal of Reproductive Medicine*, **40** (3), 171–175.

Mishriki, S.F., Law, D.J.W., Jeffery, P.J. (1990) Factors affecting the incidence of post-operative wound infection. *Journal of Hospital Infection*, **16**, 223–230.

Moffat, F.C., Deital, M., Thompson, D.A. (1982) Abdominal surgery in patients undergoing long-term peritoneal dialysis. *Surgery*, **92**, 598–604.

Morgan, H., White, B. (1983) Sleep deprivation. *Nursing Mirror*, **157** (14 Suppl.), 8–11.

Moro, M.L., Carrieri, M.P., Tozzi, A.E., Lana, S., Greco, D. (1996) Risk factors for surgical wound infections in clean surgery: a multicentre study. Italian PRINOS Study Group. *Annals of Italian Chirugia*, **67** (1), 13–19.

Morrison, P., Bernard, P. (1989) Students' and trained nurses' perceptions of their own interpersonal skills: a report and comparison. *Journal of Advanced Nursing*, **14**, 321–329.

Morrison, R. (1992) Diagnosing spiritual pain in patients. *Nursing Standard*, **6** (25), 36–38.

Moseley, L.H., Finseth, F., Goody, M. (1978) Nicotine and its effects on wound healing. *Plastic and Reconstructive Surgery*, **92**, 570–575.

Mullholland, J.H., Wright, A.M., Vinci, V., Shafiroff, B. (1943) Protein metabolism and bedsores. *Annals of Surgery*, **118**, 1015–1023.

Narayanasamy, A. (1996) Spiritual care of chronically ill patients. *British Journal of Nursing*, **5** (7), 411–416.

Nightingale, F. (1859) (repr. 1974) *Notes on Nursing, What it is and What it is not.* Blackie & Son, Glasgow and London.

Nyatanga, B. (1997) Psychosocial theories of patient non-compliance. *Professional Nurse*, **12** (5), 331–334.

Nylen, B., Wallenius, G. (1961) Protein loss via exudation from burns and granulating wound surfaces. *Acta Chirurgica Scandinavica*, **122**, 97–100.

O'Brien, M.E. (1982) Religious faith and adjustment to long-term dialysis. *Journal of Religion and Health*, **21**, 68.

Older, M.W.J., Edwards, D., Dickerson, J.W.T. (1980) A nutrient survey in elderly women with femoral neck fracture. *British Journal of Surgery*, **67**, 884.

Parsons, E.P. (1992) Cultural aspects of pain. *Surgical Nurse*, **5** (2), 14–16.

Parsons, G. (1994) The benefits of relaxation in the control of pain. *Nursing Times*, **90** (19), 11–12.

Patterson, B.M., Cornell, C.N., Carbone, B., Levine, B., Chapman, D. (1992) Protein depletion and metabolic stress in elderly patients who have a fracture of the hip. *Journal of Bone & Joint Surgery (American)*, **74** (2), 251–260.

Payman, B.C., Dampier, S.E., Hawthorn, P.J. (1989) Post-operative temperature and infection in patients undergoing general surgery. *Journal of Advanced Nursing*, **14**, 198–202.

Peck, M. (1987) *The Different Drum: Community Making and Peace*. Simon & Schuster, New York.

Pedley, H. (1996) The nurse's role in pain assessment and management in a coronary care unit. *Intensive and Critical Care Nursing*, **12**, 254–260.

Penfold, P., Crowther, S. (1989) Causes and management of neglected diet in the elderly. *Care of the Elderly*, **1** (1), 20–22.

Pinchkofsky-Devin, G.D., Kaminski, M.V. (1986) Correlation of pressure sores and nutritional status. *Journal of American Geriatric Society*, **34**, 435–440.

Pracek, J.T., Patterson, D.R., Montgomery, B.K., Heimbach, D.M. (1995) Pain, coping and adjustments in patients with burns: preliminary findings from a prospective study. *Journal of Pain and Symptom Management*, **10** (6), 446–455.

Radcliffe, S. (1993) Pre-operative information: the role of the ward nurse. *British Journal of Nursing*, **2** (6), 305–309.

Robinson, S., Falcone, R.E., Nappi, J.F. (1990) The effect of cisplatin on wound bursting strength in the rat. *Wounds*, **2** (3), 116–119.

Royal College of Surgeons and College of Anaesthetists (1990) *Commission on the Provision of Surgical Services: Report of the Working Party on Pain after Surgery*. Royal College of Surgeons and College of Anaesthetists, London.

Salmela, R.J., Ahonen, J. (1981) The effect of methylprednisolone and vitamin A on wound healing. *Acta Chirurgica Scandinavica*, **147**, 307–311.

Sassler, A.M., Esclamado, RM, Wolf, G.T. (1995) Surgery after organ preservation therapy. *Archives of Otolaryngology – Head and Neck Surgery*, **121** (2), 162–165.

Senter, H., Pringle, A. (1985) *How Wounds Heal*. Calmic Medical Division of the Wellcome Foundation.

Shipes, E. (1987) Psycho-social issues, the person with an ostomy. *Nursing Clinics of North America*, **22** (2), 291–302.

Siana, J.E., Frankild, S., Gottrup, F. (1992) The effect of smoking on tissue function. *Journal of Wound Care*, **1** (2), 37–41.

Simons, W., Malaber, R. (1995) Assessing pain in elderly patients who cannot respond verbally. *Journal of Advanced Nursing*, **22** (4), 663–669.

Simsen, B. (1986) The spiritual dimension. *Nursing Times*, **82** (48), 41–42.

Sitton-Kent, L., Gilchrist, B. (1993) The intake of nutrients by hospitalised pensioners with chronic wounds. *Journal of Advanced Nursing*, **18**, 1962–1967.

Sloman, R., Brown, P., Aldana, E., Chee, E. (1994) The use of relaxation for the promotion of comfort and pain relief in persons with advanced cancer. *Contemporary Nurse*, **3** (1), 6–12.

Smith, S. (1992) Tiresome healing. *Nursing Times*, **88** (36), 24–26.

Stead, W. (1985) One awake, all awake! *Nursing Mirror*, **160** (16), 20–21.

Stepnick, A., Perry, T. (1992) Preventing spiritual distress. *Journal of Psychosocial Nursing*, **30** (1), 17–24.

Stockwell, F. (1972) *The Unpopular Patient* Royal College of Nursing, London.

Stronge, J. (1984) Principles of wound care. *Nursing*, **2** (26 Suppl.), 7–10.

Stubbs, L. (1989) Taste changes in cancer patients. *Nursing Times*, **85** (3), 49–50.

Sutherland, A.B. (1985) Nutrition and general factors influencing infection in burns. *Journal of Hospital Infection*, **6** (Suppl. B), 31–42.

Taube, M., Elliot, P., Ellis, H. (1981) Jaundice and wound healing – a tissue culture study. *British Journal of Experimental Pathology*, **62**, 227–231.

Taylor, C.M., Cress, S.S. (1987) *Nursing Diagnosis Cards*. Springhouse Corporation, Pennsylvania.

Taylor, L.J. (1978) An evaluation of handwashing techniques, parts 1 & 2. *Nursing Times*, **74** (2), 54 & **74** (3), 108–110.

Taylor, L.K., Kuttler, K.L., Parks, T.A., Milton, D. (1998) The effect of music in the post-anaesthesia care unit on pain levels in women who have had abdominal hysterectomies. *Journal of Perianesthesia Nursing*, **13** (2), 88–94.

Tkatch, L., Rapin, C.H., Rizzoli, R., Slosman, D., Nydegger, V., Bonjour, J.P. (1992) Benefits of oral protein supplementation in elderly patients with fracture of the proximal femur. *Journal of the American College of Nutritionists*, **11** (5), 519–525.

Tschudin, V. (1991) Just four questions. *Nursing Times*, **87** (39), 46–47.

Volicer, B.J., Bohannon, M.W. (1975) A hospital stress rating scale. *Nursing Research*, **24**, 352–359.

Walker, B.B. (1972) The postsurgery heart patient: amount of uninterrupted time for sleep and rest during the first, second and third postoperative days in a teaching hospital. *Nursing Research*, **21** (2), 164–169.

Ward, S.E., Berry, P.E., Misiewicz, H. (1996) Concerns about analgesics among patients and family caregivers in a hospice setting. *Research in Nursing & Health*, **19** (3), 205–211.

Wilkinson, S. (1992a) Good communication in cancer nursing. *Nursing Standard*, **7** (9), 35–39.

Wilkinson, S. (1992b) Confusions and challenges. *Nursing Times*, **88** (35), 24–28.

Woods, N. (1972) Patterns of sleep in post-cardiotomy patients. *Nursing Research*, **21**, 347–352.

Yates, P., Dewar, A., Fentiman, B. (1995) Pain: the views of elderly people living in long-term residential care settings. *Journal of Advanced Nursing*, **21** (4), 667–674.

Zainal, G. (1995) Nutritional demands. *Nursing Times*, **91** (38), 57–59.

Zigmond, A.S., Snaith, R.P. (1983) The hospital anxiety and depression scale. *Acta Psychiatrica Scandinavica*, **67**, 361–370.

Chapter 3
General Principles of Wound Management

3.1 INTRODUCTION

This section will discuss, in broad detail, the general principles of wound management. Specific care of chronic and acute wounds will be considered in later chapters. The products mentioned in this chapter will be described in more detail in Chapter 4.

The ability to make an accurate assessment of a wound is an important nursing skill. It should be carried out in conjunction with an assessment of the patient as discussed in Chapter 2. The aim of the assessment is two-fold: (1) it will provide baseline information on the state of the wound so that progress can be monitored; (2) it will also ensure that an appropriate selection of wound management products is made. The management of the different types of wounds will be discussed.

There are several factors to consider when assessing a wound. They are:

(1) The wound classification.
(2) The depth of the wound.
(3) The shape and size of the wound.
(4) The amount of wound exudate.
(5) The position of the wound.
(6) Wound appearance.
(7) The environment of care.

3.2 PLANNING WOUND CARE

3.2.1 Wound classification

Wounds can be classified as chronic, acute and postoperative wounds.

Chronic wounds have been described by Fowler (1990) as being of long duration or frequent recurrence. Typical examples are pressure sores and leg ulcers. Patients may have multifactorial problems which affect their ability to heal their wounds.

Acute wounds are usually traumatic wounds. They may be cuts, abrasions, lacerations, burns or other traumatic wounds. They usually respond rapidly to treatment and heal without complication.

Postoperative wounds are intentional acute wounds. They may be healing by first intention, where the skin edges are held in approximation. Sutures, clips or tape may be used. Some surgical wounds are left open to heal by second intention, usually to allow drainage of infected material. Donor sites are also open wounds.

Whatever the type of wound the healing process is the same. However, there may be related factors to be considered when managing each of these types of wounds, such as the relief of pressure for pressure sores. The care of chronic wounds will be considered in Chapter 5 and of acute wounds in Chapter 6.

3.2.2 The description of wounds according to depth

This type of classification is widely used in the USA, but generally only used to describe burns or, occasionally, pressure sores in the UK.

Wounds are described in relation to the tissues which are damaged or destroyed. Figure 3.1 illustrates the different depths of tissue damage.

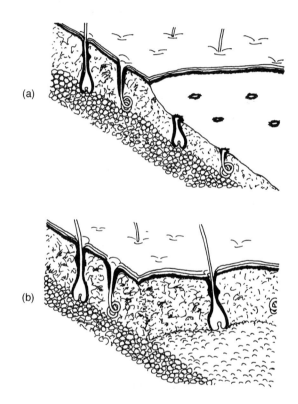

(a)

(b)

Fig. 3.1   The degree of tissue damage in wounds of differing depth. (a) Partial-thickness wound: islets of living epithelium remain around hair shafts and sweat ducts; (b) full-thickness wound: no living epithelia remain in the injured area.

Erosion is the term used to describe the loss of one or two layers of epithelial cells. There is no depth to this type of wound.

Superficial wounds are wounds where the epidermis has been damaged.

A partial-thickness wound is when the epithelium and part of the dermis is destroyed. Hair follicles and sweat glands are only partially damaged. This type of wound is sometimes sub-divided into partial-thickness and deep-partial-thickness wounds. When these wounds have a large surface area, hair follicles and sweat glands produce epithelial cells during the stage of epithelialisation which form islets of cells on the wound surface, thus speeding the healing process.

Full-thickness wounds have all of the epidermis and dermis destroyed. Deeper tissues such as muscle or bone may also be involved. Healing may take longer to establish in these wounds.

3.2.3 The shape and size of the wound

The size and shape of a wound may alter during the healing process. In the early stages, as necrotic tissue and/or slough are removed, the wound appears to increase in size. This is because the true extent of the wound was masked by the necrotic tissue. Monitoring of wound shape is important to aid in dressing selection. A cavity wound requires a different dressing to a shallow wound. Some dressings are not appropriate for use if there is a sinus present. Accurate nursing records are essential for monitoring progress. Wound measurement is addressed in Section 3.3 of this chapter.

3.2.4 The amount of wound exudate

The amount of wound exudate varies during the healing process. There is considerable exudate at the inflammatory stage and very little at epithelialisation. A copious exudate may indicate a prolonged inflammatory stage or infection. It also affects dressing selection as a very absorbent dressing may be necessary. Maceration of the surrounding skin may occur if a dressing is used that cannot cope with the level of exudate (see Plate 2).

3.2.5 The position of the wound

The position of a wound should be noted as part of the assessment. It may be an indication of potential problems, such as risk of contamination in wounds in the sacral region, or problems of mobility caused by wounds on the foot. Another aspect is the fact that a dressing may stay in place very well on one part of the body but not on another.

3.2.6 Wound appearance

The appearance of the wound gives an indication of the stage of healing that it has reached or of any complication that may be present. Open wounds or wounds healing by second intention can be categorised as:

- necrotic
- infected
- sloughy
- granulating
- epithelialising

Some wounds may be seen to have more than one category and so present as 'mixed' wounds. Before assessing a wound, the nurse should ensure that all the old dressing has been removed. Many modern dressings form a gel which may give a misleading impression of the wound unless it is first cleansed away.

Necrotic wounds (see Plate 3)

When an area of tissue becomes ischaemic for any length of time, it will die. The area may form a necrotic eschar or scab. This can be black or brown in colour. Some necrotic tissue may present as a thick slough which can be brown, grey or off-white. When assessing these wounds it is important to remember that the wound may be more extensive than is apparent. The eschar or slough masks the true size of the wound. Intervention is needed for these wounds to heal.

● *Management* ●

(1) The wound covered with a hard necrotic eschar.
The aim of management is to remove the necrotic tissue from the wound. There are a variety of ways that this can be achieved. If the necrotic tissue is beginning to separate, surgical debridement can be used. This is a very quick way of removing the eschar, but is not always the most appropriate. Wound management products, such as hydrocolloids or an amorphous hydrogel, may be used to soften and liquefy the necrotic tissue. Colin *et al.* (1996) found an amorphous hydrogel was more effective than a dextranomer paste in debriding necrotic pressure sores. Biosurgery or larvae therapy has also been used to debride necrotic eschar (Thomas *et al.*, 1996). It should be noted that as the necrotic tissue liquefies it has a very offensive odour.

(2) The wound filled with exudating necrotic tissue.
Patients find it very distressing to have a heavily exuding, offensive wound. An alginate dressing may be the most effective when there is heavy exudate. In the case of cavity wounds an alginate rope may be used. If there is a moderate exudate, either hydrocolloids or an amorphous hydrogel can be used. Hydrocolloid powder or paste which can be placed into a cavity and then covered with the hydrocolloid wafer may also be effective. Surgical debridement can be used to remove any loose necrotic tissue. A charcoal dressing can be used to help reduce odour. It can be used in conjunction with any of the above products except the hydrocolloids, which do not require a secondary dressing. Larvae therapy may also be effective in necrotic cavities.

Infected wounds (see Plate 4)

All wounds are colonised with bacteria. This does not delay healing or mean that wounds will automatically become infected. Cruse and Foord (1980) and Meers (1981) defined an infected wound as one which has a purulent discharge. Other definitions consider the host reaction. If host resistance is adequate to cope with the colonising bacteria, then no infection will occur. Altemeier (1979) proposed a formula to define this:

$$\frac{\text{Dose of bacteria} \times \text{Virulence}}{\text{Host reaction}} = \text{Probability of infection}$$

The host reaction to bacterial colonisation and the risk of infection has already been discussed in Section 2.2.1 of Chapter 2.

Cutting and Harding (1994) propose additional criteria to those discussed above. They are:

(1) Delayed healing (compared with expected rate, may be for other reasons).
(2) Discoloration: relates to wound bed.
(3) Friable granulation tissue which bleeds easily.
(4) Unexpected pain or tenderness.
(5) Pocketing or bridging at the base of the wound.
(6) Abnormal odour; this should not be confused with debriding necrotic eschar.
(7) Wound breakdown: most commonly seen in wounds healing by first intention.

Clinical signs of infection can be observed. They may vary slightly according to the bacteria causing the infection. Usually there is localised erythema or redness. It may be restricted to just one part of the wound, such as at one end of a suture line, or it may spread to a large area around the wound. Associated with the erythema is cellulitis in the adjacent tissues which will also feel hotter than the skin at a distance from the wound. It should be noted that cellulitis is not easy to observe in the presence of oedema. The colour of the exudate and the slough on the wound surface depend on the bacteria causing the infection. There is usually a heavy exudate as the body rushes extra neutrophils and macrophages to the affected area and also tries to 'wash' the bacteria away. The exudate may have an offensive odour and can be the first indication of infection.

● *Management* ●

A wound swab should be taken. This is not to prove that there is infection present, as clinical observation has already shown that there is. A swab will assist in identifying the infecting bacteria and then selecting which are the most appropriate systemic antibiotics. Wound management has to be considered in conjunction with the use of systemic antibiotics.

A variety of products may be used to manage an infected wound. Silver sulphadiazine is especially effective against *Pseudomonas aeruginosa*. Danielsen *et al.* (1997) also found Iodosorb/Iodoflex® to be effective for leg ulcers colonised with *Pseudomonas aeruginosa*. Hillstrom (1988) found Iodosorb® reduced the number of bacteria on infected wounds. Alginates are also suitable for infected wounds, but should be changed daily (Thomas, 1990). Some studies, such as Gilchrist and Reed (1988) have suggested that hydrocolloids may reduce the numbers of bacteria on the wound surface. Intrasite Gel® may be used on infected wounds (Stewart & Leaper, 1987). However, if there is copious exudate, neither of these two types of dressing is very effective.

If a wound is infected or potentially infected, but has little exudate, a different strategy may be adopted. Inadine®, a povidone-iodine tulle, may be used. The iodine is released over varying lengths of time, depending on the amount of exudate. No more than four dressings should be applied at any one time.

Infections caused by methicillin-resistant *Staphylococcus aureus* (MRSA) have to be treated rather differently from other types of infection. Guidelines have been prepared by a joint working party of the British Society for Antimicrobial Chemotherapy, the Hospital Infection Society and the Infection Control Nurses

Association (Hospital Infection Society, 1998). They recommend that mupirocin (0.5%) is applied to small infected or colonised skin lesions. It is not suitable for large wounds such as large burns. The cream should be applied daily for no more than 7–10 days. Standard infection control measures should also be in place.

Sloughy wounds (see Plate 5)

Slough is typically a white/yellow colour. It is most often found as patches on the wound surface, although it may cover large areas of the wound. It is made up of dead cells which have accumulated in the exudate. It can be related to the end of the inflammatory stage in the healing process. Neutrophils have only a short life-span and may die faster than they can be removed. Given the right environment for healing, the macrophages are usually capable of removing the slough and it disappears as healing progresses. Harding (1990) refers to a yellow fibrinous membrane that develops on the surface of some wounds. It is not stuck fast but can be easily removed. The membrane has no effect on healing and recurs if removed. He describes it as a variant on the normal.

● *Management* ●

(1) A shallow sloughy wound with low to moderate exudate.
The aim of treatment is to promote healing by ensuring that the product used as a primary dressing will provide a moist environment. This will facilitate leucocyte activity. Either hydrocolloids or an amorphous hydrogel will fulfil this requirement.
(2) A shallow sloughy wound with moderate to heavy exudate.
The wound surface should be relatively moist. The dressing should maintain this, whilst controlling the exudate. Several types of products may be used: alginates, beads, hydrocolloids or an amorphous hydrogel.
(3) A cavity filled with slough and moderate to low exudate.
The main aim is to assist in liquefying the slough to promote its removal. An amorphous hydrogel, or hydrocolloid pastes and wafers, may be used.
(4) A cavity filled with slough and a heavy to moderate exudate.
These types of wounds sometimes have copious amounts of exudate as the slough liquefies. Initially this may cause concern, but usually granulation tissue will rapidly appear and the amount of exudate will reduce. In these circumstances, alginate rope or ribbon or a hydrofibre rope is usually the most effective way of filling the cavity and absorbing the exudate.

When there is less copious exudate a range of dressings can be used, alginate rope or ribbon, beads, amorphous hydrogel or hydrocolloid paste and wafers.

Granulating wounds (see Plate 6)

Granulation tissue was first described by John Hunter in 1786. It relates quite well to the stage of reconstruction in the healing process. The wound colour is red. The tops of the capillary loops cause the surface to look granular, hence the name. It should be remembered that the walls of the capillary loops are very thin and easily damaged, which explains why these wounds bleed easily. Regular, careful measurement will show a reduction in wound volume as the cavity fills with new tissue and contracts inwards.

● *Management* ●

(1) A shallow granulating wound with low to moderate exudate.
These wounds require very little healing as there is little cavity to fill with granulation tissue. A moist environment will speed the progress to epithelialisation. A range of products may be used: flat foam dressings, hydrocolloids, hydrogels or semi-permeable films.

(2) A shallow granulating wound with moderate to high exudate.
The amount of exudate is usually less in these wounds than in necrotic, infected or sloughy wounds. The types of dressing that may be used include: alginates, hydrocellular foams, hydrogels and hydrocolloids.

(3) A cavity wound filled with granulation tissue.
The selection of a suitable product depends upon the shape of the cavity and whether any undermining or sinuses are present. For irregular cavities without sinus formation, a cavity foam dressing such as Cavi-Care® may be used, particularly on very large surgical wounds. Other dressings which may be used include alginate rope or ribbon, foam cavity fillers, such as Allevyn® cavity wound, amorphous hydrogels and hydrocolloid paste and wafers. The selection of these dressings depends on the degree of exudate.

(4) A wound with overgranulation or exuberant granulation tissue.
Occasionally granulation tissue continues to be laid down when a cavity is filled. The granulation tissue stands proud of the rest of the skin. This has been described as exuberant granulation, hypertrophic granulation tissue and also overgranulation. It poses a problem because it prevents epithelial cells from spreading across the wound. Although it has not often been documented, there seems to be a standardised treatment for overgranulation – the use of silver nitrate sticks. They have a caustic effect, thus destroying the proud tissue. Terra-Cortril® cream has also been used. No research has been carried out into the use of either of these two products for this purpose. Harris and Rolstad (1993) have investigated an alternative solution of using a flat foam dressing. In a study of 15 wounds they found that the foam dressing significantly reduced the levels of exuberant granulation tissue. Cassino *et al.* (1998) found that a hydrocellular foam dressing was also effective. The use of these types of dressings is much less traumatic than the use of silver nitrate sticks and can readily be utilised by nurses in any healthcare setting.

Epithelialising (see Plate 7)

As the epithelia at the wound margins start to divide rapidly, the margin becomes slightly raised and has a bluey-pink colour. As the epithelia spread across the wound surface, the margin flattens. The new epithelial tissue is a pinky-white colour.

In shallow wounds with a large surface area, islets of epithelialisation may be seen. The progress of epithelialisation may be easily identified as the new cells are a different colour from those of the surrounding tissue.

● *Management* ●

(1) A shallow epithelialising wound with low to moderate exudate.
Maintenance of a moist environment and protection of the fragile epithelial tissue are the main aims when choosing a dressing. Suitable dressings include foams, films, hydrocolloids and hydrogels.
(2) A shallow epithelialising wound with moderate to heavy exudate.
The aim in treating this type of wound is to control the exudate whilst protecting the wound. A variety of dressings can be used: alginates, foams, hydrocolloids and hydrogels.

Care of the skin around the wound

Little attention has been given to the need to care for the skin around a wound. Very often it will be fragile and even malnourished. A range of problems can arise:

(1) Trauma to the skin, particularly from frequent removal of adhesive tapes. Fragile skin may even tear.
(2) Allergy to the tape or dressing (contact dermatitis), which usually manifests itself as erythema or redness where it was applied. In severe cases there may also be blistering. It is important to differentiate between contact dermatitis and irritant dermatitis. The latter may occur if there is persistent heavy exudate which is poorly controlled either by using a dressing of insufficient absorbency or by not changing the dressing when necessary. Plates 8 and 9 demonstrate the difference very clearly. Plate 8 shows an allergic reaction to a dressing where the erythema is confined to the area covered by the dressing. Plate 9 shows severe irritant dermatitis caused by uncontrolled exudate over a long period of time in a patient who refused to wear compression bandages for venous ulceration.
(3) Dryness and flakiness of the skin, particularly when bandages are used in conjunction with the dressing. This problem is only likely to occur in chronic wounds where it is not always possible to maintain usual bathing routines. As a result, skin scales are not washed away and collect on the area around the wound.

● *Management* ●

When assessing the wound and planning appropriate care, it is important to assess and monitor the skin around the wound. Little research has been carried out in this area. A study by Dealey (1992) showed the benefits of using protective skin wipes. Originally developed to be used around stoma sites, they are widely used in wound care in the USA. This study showed the benefits of using skin wipes, both to protect fragile skin and when skin trauma and/or allergy had occurred. Plate 10 shows a patient with severe oedema and fragile skin who had two small ulcerations on her leg. Her skin was protected with a skin wipe and a thin hydrocolloid applied. Plate 11 shows the leg a week later. One ulcer has healed and the skin has remained intact. Plates 12 and 13 show a patient with a superficial pressure sore who had known allergies to film, foam and hydrocolloid dressings. The protective wipe was applied to the skin under a film dressing and the sore was virtually healed within a week. The study clearly demonstrates the benefits of protecting the skin in this way.

Dryness of the skin is more difficult to combat. Emollients can help, but may affect dressing retention. Where it is practicable, bathing or showering using emollients will help to remove skin scales. Creams can also be applied to the affected area avoiding the wound margins.

There is need for further research into this aspect of wound care.

3.2.7 The environment of care

Consideration must be given to the environment in which care is to be given. Harding (1992) proposed a wound-healing matrix which includes consideration of the environment and carer. The management of a wound can be affected by the circumstances of the patient. For example, the timing of a dressing change may not be important for a patient in hospital. However, for a patient at home, perhaps a young mother with children to get to school, timing may be critical. Flexibility may be important for a patient with a longstanding wound who has to return to work. It may be helpful to arrange for the occupational health nurse in the patient's place of employment to carry out the dressing change, thus reducing the frequency of clinic attendance. Not all wound management products are available in the community. Hospital nurses need to ensure that the product selected can be continued after discharge home. If a non-skilled person is to provide some of the wound care for a patient, adequate time must be allowed for teaching the individual appropriate routines. Adequate monitoring of care must also be established.

3.2.8 Evaluating the wound

In order to judge the progress of a wound, it is essential to make objective measurements on initial assessment, and to repeat at regular intervals. Nursing charts can provide a useful framework. Figure 3.2 is an example of an assessment sheet that could be used to record the initial assessment of a wound. Some form of measurement should be incorporated into the assessment. Measurement is discussed in more detail in Section 3.3. Other charts can incorporate ongoing evaluation and are particularly relevant to surgical wounds (see Chapter 6).]

If a wound fails to heal or make progress then it is helpful to have a checklist to see if any related factors have been missed. This can be presented in the form of a flow chart such as Table 3.1.

If this fails to highlight any problem, consider the management of the wound. How long has the dressing been used? No improvement may be seen for up to two weeks with chronic wounds. A common problem is the lack of continuity in management. The type of dressing being altered every shift according to the individual whim of the nurse on duty. Rundgren *et al.* (1990) followed the progress of 101 patients with a variety of wounds over a five-month period. They found that from week to week about 30% of the patients were receiving a different treatment. Also that 65% of the wounds did not heal even though they were having treatment for the whole of the study period. They concluded that this lack of continuity was

TISSUE VIABILITY DEPARTMENT
OPEN WOUND ASSESSMENT CHART

Type of Wound	
How long has wound been open?	
Location	
General patient factors which may delay healing. (e.g. malnourished, diabetic, chronic infection, medication)	
Allergies to wound care products	
Previous treatments used.	
Pressure Relieving Equipment (e.g. pressure relieving bed, cushion)	

Wound Factors Date:				
Wound Classification healthy granulation epithelialisation slough black/brown necrotic tissue infected				
Exudate - Amount				
Odour offensive/some/none				
Wound Dimensions length width depth				
Wound Photographed?				
Pain (Site) at wound site elsewhere (specify)				
Pain (frequency) continuous/intermittent/ only at dressing changes/ at night/none				
Pain (severity) 0 = none 10 = excruciating				
Condition of surrounding skin (fragile, reddened, dry etc)				
Refer to CNS in Tissue Y/N **Viability** Date				
Wound Assessed by:				
Next Review date:				

Fig. 3.2 Wound assessment form.

related to poor documentation, impatience and a lack of understanding of the healing process.

3.2.9 Evaluating the dressing

Nurses should be prepared to evaluate objectively the dressings they use. This is particularly important if they are using new dressings, although traditional dressings

Table 3.1 Flow chart: failure to heal.

Does the patient appear anxious?	→ **YES** →	Encourage patient to express anxieties
↓ **NO** ↓		
Is there oedema or ischaemia around wound site? (especially leg ulcers?	→ **YES** →	Correct positioning of limbs. Use compression (in oedema); medical opinion
↓ **NO** ↓		
Are there signs of infection – urinary tract, chest, wound?	→ **YES** →	Culture of bacteria, medical opinion; systemic antibiotics
↓ **NO** ↓		
Has patient reduced nutritional status?	→ **YES** →	Cause? Improve nutritional intake
↓ **NO** ↓		
Has patient's general condition deteriorated? (disease-related)	→ **YES** →	Medical opinion
↓ **NO** ↓		
Is patient having sufficient sleep?	→ **NO** →	Cause? Medical opinion? Night sedation or analgesia?
↓ **YES**		

should not be exempt from reappraisal. When evaluating a dressing, various aspects need to be considered:

(1) Patient comfort.
(2) Ease of application.
(3) Effectiveness.
(4) Cost.

Patient comfort is of primary importance for any wound management product. It can be very distressing for patients when the application of a dressing is painful. Eusol is a well known example of a lotion which causes pain on application (see Chapter 4). Other products may adhere to the wound and cause discomfort to patients when they move, and pain when the dressing is removed. A dressing which fails to provide sufficient absorbency and allows leakage of exudate can cause considerable inconvenience, as well as promoting feelings of insecurity in the patient.

Although different nurses may carry out the dressing, the patient is always present. Any evaluation should involve the patient. Many like to take an interest and can provide valuable information on new products.

Ease of application means that a dressing can be applied effectively and so stay in place. When using any new product, it may take a little practice to develop the most effective method of application. The nurse should be prepared to try a dressing over a period of time on a variety of wounds (unless contraindicated) and on different parts of the body. This will allow a more comprehensive evaluation.

Effectiveness is most important. If a product does not promote healing, then it does not matter if it is comfortable or easy to apply. Before a product becomes available for general use, it should have undergone stringent laboratory tests to check for safety. Marks (1986) also advocates the use of models of wound healing. He rightly states that it is extremely difficult to conduct good clinical trials as there can be so many variables. Hunt (1983) considered the additional difficulties of undertaking a clinical nursing trial. She suggested that they included a lack of control over the admission and discharge of patients, staffing patterns and the large numbers of nurses involved in patient care and the variations in patterns of care within any health authority.

If nurses are to evaluate the effectiveness of any dressing they use, they need to be aware of any research which has been published. They also need to be able to analyse it in order to ascertain its value. The NHS Executive (1998) has produced useful guidelines on how to appraise a piece of research critically. MacAuley *et al.* (1998) found the use of a formal assessment tool was more effective than free appraisal amongst 243 general practitioners.

Cost is seen as an important factor in all aspects of care. It should be considered when evaluating any dressing. However, not only the unit cost is relevant. The overall costs should be considered. One example is a study by Thomas and Tucker (1989) who compared the use of paraffin tulle with that of an alginate (Sorbsan®) and found a reduced overall cost using Sorbsan® despite the fact that the unit cost is greater than that of tulle. All the implications of the cost of healing will be considered in Chapter 9.

3.3 WOUND MEASUREMENT

This section considers the various ways that a measurement of a wound may be made. Some of them are not really appropriate for use in busy areas, but may have a value in a small-scale research study. Others are very expensive and outside the pocket of most nurses.

Whatever measurement is used, it should be done on a regular basis, the frequency depending on the type of wound. Chronic wounds should be measured every 2–4 weeks – little change is likely to be seen by more frequent measurement; however, acute wounds progress much more rapidly, and measurement should be done at each dressing change.

Regular measurement will enable some sort of monitoring of the rate of healing. The final part of this section will look at some of the mathematical methods for measuring the rate of healing, enabling comparison between wounds and different methods of management.

3.3.1 Simple measurement

The very simplest method of measuring a wound is to measure it at its greatest length and breadth and to measure the depth if appropriate. If a wound is a relatively regular shape such as the example shown in Fig. 3.3, then this can be a fairly successful method. It is also likely to be more accurate if the wound edges are marked to indicate the measurement points. A probe can be used if the wound is a very irregular shape or has sinus formation.

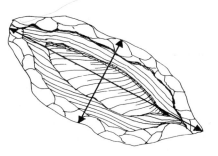

Fig. 3.3 Measurement of a regular-shaped wound.

There are several drawbacks to using this type of measurement. The accuracy may be rather doubtful if it is done by a great many people. The more people involved, the greater the risk of the measurement not being on the same spot each time. It is fair to state that even if the same person does the measurement each time, it still may not be replicated accurately. This is known as sampling error. If necrotic tissue or slough is present, the true wound size will become apparent as debridement occurs. Wound measurement will show that the wound has increased in size and can give a misleading picture of wound progress. Measurement gives no indication of wound appearance.

● *Overall comment* ●

Measurement is best used on small, surgically induced cavities which are regular in shape and should heal rapidly. More comprehensive data would be obtained if used in conjunction with a nursing chart such as that shown in Fig. 3.2.

3.3.2 Wound tracing

Another frequently used system is that of tracing a wound. A variety of materials may be used, the commonest being acetate paper. One presentation of acetate paper is the lesion measure, samples of which are supplied by several dressing manufacturers. They are usually fairly small sheets with a series of circles on them.

The centre circle is 1 cm in diameter and is surrounded by concentric circles which increase in size by 2 cm increments. This gives some estimate of measurement in the tracing.

The surface area of a wound can be calculated quite accurately by placing the tracing over squared paper and counting the number of whole squares. Successive tracings can be compared to show any difference in wound size. If necrotic tissue or slough is present then an initial increase in size will occur as debridement progresses. As with wound measurement, the tracing will show the increase in size without any explanation as it does not provide information on wound appearance or depth. There are also the same risks of inaccuracy. Anthony (1993) describes some of the discrepancies found with this method. Vowden (1995) discusses some of the ways that the surface area of a wound can be calculated and showed how they can produce different results for the same wound.

A more sophisticated version of tracing is the use of paper that can be used to convert surface area to weight. A tracing of the wound is made and the shape cut out. This wound shape is then weighed. Likely sampling errors in this method include altering the size/shape of the wound when cutting the paper.

If the acetate sheet is placed in direct contact with the wound it will need cleansing with alcohol spray or similar. Some centres use plastic bags so the underside can be discarded and the side with the tracing retained. Some acetates are provided with disposable backing paper.

● *Overall comment* ●

Tracing is best used on fairly straightforward shallow wounds. Ideally it should be used in combination with an assessment chart, e.g. Fig. 3.2.

3.3.3 Photography

The old adage 'a picture is worth a thousand words' may not be strictly true in relation to photographs of wounds, but photography does address some of the criticisms of the previous methods. A photograph provides clear evidence of the appearance of a wound and some suggestion of its size. Myers and Cherry (1984) incorporated a rule in their photographs to provide a scale. Minns and Whittle (1992) describe an aluminium frame attachment to a Polaroid camera which has graduated scales to allow calculation of wound size. Polaroid has a Gridfilm® which superimposes a grid over the wound on the photograph and can be used to calculate wound area (Wallace, 1994). When managing chronic wounds, regular photographs can provide real encouragement to both patients and carers.

There are problems with photographs as a record of wound progress. The depth of a wound is not demonstrated in a photograph as it does not accurately record wounds on curved surfaces. Not all nurses have access to a camera. It may be possible to obtain one on a short-term loan if a dressing trial is being undertaken.

Several factors need to be considered if the purchase of a camera is planned.

● Who will pay for films and developing?
● Is the proposed camera capable of taking close-up pictures?

- Who will be using the camera?
- How can pictures be taken from the same angle and distance each time?
- How can individual patients be identified if using a film with large numbers of exposures?

A Polaroid camera may resolve some of these problems – if a photograph is no good, another can be taken immediately. Whilst the quality may not be as good as more powerful cameras, it is adequate for most needs, especially if a lightlock lens is used to enable close-ups.

● *Overall comment* ●

Photographs provide good visual evidence of wound appearance. If a camera is not easily available, photography is best only considered for complicated or unusual wounds. It would be helpful to use some form of wound measurement, such as a scale bar, with the photographs.

3.3.4 Stereophotogrammetry

Stereophotogrammetry is a system which was developed to obtain measurement of the volume of a wound. It does this by providing a three-dimensional picture from two photographs taken simultaneously from different angles. The image thus obtained can be measured. Bulstrode *et al.* (1986) used this method in conjunction with a metrograph and a computer. Goode (1990) considers this method to be far superior to other methods such as tracing or photography. Frantz and Johnson (1992) have developed a method of using stereophotogrammetry with computerised image analysis which they have found to be suitable for clinical trials.

Several drawbacks must be considered. It is highly unlikely that many nurses would have access to such equipment. Special training or the availability of trained personnel would also be necessary. It takes about 20 minutes to carry out the procedure. When taking images on a one-off basis, no particular position or point is necessary. However, if a series of pictures is required, the same position should be reproduced each time.

● *Overall comment* ●

Whilst it is interesting to be aware of such equipment, it is not appropriate for everyday use.

3.3.5 Computerised systems of wound measurement

In recent years the development of computer imaging has made dramatic strides. It is used in many ways from providing interior 'views' of a building to giving images of parts of the human body. The potential is enormous: van Riet Paap *et al.* (1991) describe a digital image analysis system made up of a video attached to a computer. The image can be reproduced from the same position each time and can be used on wounds of any size. Digital cameras are now readily available and allow transfer of the image to computer.

A fairly new method involves the use of structured light. Plassmann *et al.* (1993) describe how a camera is connected to an image-processing computer which scans the wound which is bathed in light. The computer is able to calculate the wound dimensions. Ongoing studies have found that this method has also been able to measure wound appearance, and correctly identified 90% of infected wounds and 73% of non-infected wounds (Plassman, 1998). It is unable to measure deep wounds or wounds which change shape.

Another computer program is able to calculate the surface area of a wound. First, it makes a photocopy of a tracing of the wound from which it makes the necessary calculation. The use of computers is still limited for most nurses. As this increases, more nurses will become computer literate and confident in managing some of the sophisticated programs available.

● *Overall comment* ●

These are exciting developments, but only available to limited numbers at present.

3.3.6 Measuring the rate of healing

Several researchers have used some of the methods of wound measurement to develop a system for measuring healing. This enables the researcher to compare the healing rate of wounds of different sizes. Although they are not used routinely in many areas, they are of interest.

Gowland-Hopkins and Jamieson (1983) devised a formula to describe the healing rate using wound tracings. The tracings gave information about the original wound circumference, the current wound circumference and the size of the healed area. A formula then calculated the radius of the healed area. Gilman (1990) also proposed a formula based on the linear advance of the wound circumference towards the centre of the wound. He suggested that this could be used on wounds of differing size and would permit an unbiased comparison of the rates of healing.

Resch *et al.* (1988) put forward a different way of measuring healing rates of pressure sores. They used an alginate compound, commonly used to take dental impressions, to make a mould of a wound. The mould could subsequently be weighed and the volume calculated. The mould also provided a visual record of the shape of the wound. A series of moulds would show the reduction (if any) in size and volume, thus showing the healing rate. They considered that this method was particularly useful on irregularly shaped wounds which are very difficult to measure in other ways.

Marks *et al.* (1983) observed the rates of healing of 40 laparotomy wounds healing by second intention and 29 pilonidal sinus excisions. The linear regression of healing time against wound size was calculated. Wound size was considered to be the size of the width or depth of the wound, whichever was the greater. A 'predicted' healing time was then calculated for each type of wound. Thus any laparotomy wound or pilonidal sinus excision could be measured and expected healing time calculated. Early indication of healing problems could be obtained if the wound failed to maintain the predicted rate of healing. This type of calculation is useful only for regular-shaped surgical wounds which would be expected to heal without complication.

● *Overall comment* ●

These types of measurement are not likely to be used in general nursing care.

3.3.7 Conclusions

Wound measurement is an important aspect of the assessment and evaluation process. For the vast majority of wounds, simple operations such as measuring or tracing a wound are perfectly satisfactory. A series of measurements can be used to give some idea of the rate of healing. It may be useful to use one of the methods of calculating healing rates, if undertaking clinical trials of a specific wound management product. For large-scale studies access to a computer is usually necessary as manual calculations of large numbers is very time consuming.

REFERENCES

Altemeier, W.A. (1979) Principles in the management of traumatic wounds and in infection control. *Bulletin of New York Academy of Medicine*, **55** (2), 123–138.

Anthony, D. (1993) The assessment of the skin of the elderly patient with specific reference to decubitus ulcers and incontinence dermatitis. *Journal of Tissue Viability*, **3** (3), 85–93, 99.

Bulstrode, C.J.K., Goode, A.W., Scott, P.J. (1986) Stereophotogrammetry for measuring rates of cutaneous healing: a comparison with conventional techniques. *Clinical Science*, **71**, 437–443.

Cassino, R., Ricci, E., Carusone, A., Mercanti, A. (1998) The successful treatment of hypergranulating wounds using a hydrocellular dressing, in (eds) Leaper, D., Cherry, G., Cockbill, S., Dealey, C., Flanagan, M., Hofman, D., *et al.*, *Proceedings of the EWMA/Journal of Wound Care Spring Conference*. Macmillan Magazines Ltd, London.

Colin, D., Kurring, P.A., Quinlan, D., Yvon, C. (1996) The clinical investigation of an amorphous hydrogel compared with a dextranomer paste dressing in the management of sloughy pressure sores, in (eds) Cherry, G., Gottrup, F., Lawrence, J.C., Moffatt, C.J., Turner, T.D., *Proceedings of the 5th European Conference on Advances in Wound Management*. Macmillan Magazines Ltd, London.

Cruse, P.J.E., Foord, R. (1980) The epidemiology of wound infection. *Surgical Clinics of North America*, **60** (1), 27–40.

Cutting, K., Harding, K.G. (1994) Criteria for identifying wound infection. *Journal of Wound Care*, **3** (4), 198–201.

Danielsen, L., Cherry, G., Harding, K., Rollman, O. (1997) Use of Iodosorb/Iodoflex on venous leg ulcer colonised with *Pseudomonas aeruginosa*, in (eds) Leaper, D.J., Cherry, G., Dealey, C., Lawrence, J.C., Turner, T.D., *Proceedings of the 6th European Conference on Advances in Wound Management*. Macmillan Magazines Ltd, London.

Dealey, C. (1992) Using protective skin wipes under adhesive tapes. *Journal of Wound Care*, **1** (2), 19–22.

Fowler, E. (1990) Chronic wounds: an overview, in (ed) Krasner, D., *Chronic Wound Care: A Clinical Sourcebook for Healthcare Professionals*. Health Management Publications Inc., King of Prussia, Pennsylvania.

Frantz, R.A., Johnson, D.A. (1992) Stereophotography and computerised image analysis: a three-dimensional method of measuring wound healing. *Wounds*, **4** (2), 58–63.

Gilchrist, B., Reed, C. (1988) The bacteriology of leg ulcers under occlusive dressings, in (ed) Ryan, T.J., *Beyond Occlusion: Wound Care Proceedings*. Royal Society of Medicine, London.

Gilman, T.H. (1990) Parameter for measurement of wound closure. *Wounds*, **2** (3), 95–101.

Goode, A.W. (1990) Metabolic basis of wound healing, in (ed) Bader, D., *Pressure Sores – Clinical Practice and Scientific Approach*. Macmillan Press, London.

Gowland-Hopkins, N.F., Jamieson, C.W. (1983) Antibiotic concentrations in the exudate of venous ulcers: the prediction of the healing rate. *British Journal of Surgery*, **70**, 532–534.

Harding, K.G. (1990) Wound care: putting theory into practice, in (ed) Krasner, D., *Chronic Wound Care: A Clinical Sourcebook for Healthcare Professionals*. Health Management Publications Inc., King of Prussia, Pennsylvania.

Harding, K.G. (1992) The wound-healing matrix. *Journal of Wound Care*, **1** (3), 40–44.

Harris, A., Rolstad, B.S. (1993) Hypergranulation tissue: a non-traumatic method of management, in (eds) Harding, K.G., Cherry, G., Dealey, C., Turner, T.D., *Proceedings of the 2nd European Conference on Advances in Wound Management*. Macmillan Magazines Ltd, London.

Hillstrom, L. (1988) Iodosorb compared to standard treatment in chronic venous leg ulcers – a multicentre trial. *Acta Chirurgica Scandinavica*, Suppl. 554, 53–56.

Hospital Infection Society (1998) Revised guidelines for the control of methicillin-resistant *Staphylococcus aureus* infection in hospitals. *Journal of Hospital Infection*, **39**, 253–290.

Hunt, J. (1983) Product evaluation. *Nursing*, **2** (12 Suppl.), 6–7.

MacAuley, D., McCrum, E., Brown, C. (1998) Randomised controlled trial of the READER method of critical appraisal in general practice. *British Medical Journal*, **316**, 1134–1137.

Marks, J., Hughes, L.E., Harding, K.G., Campbell, H., Ribeiro, C.D. (1983) Prediction of healing time as an aid to the management of open granulating wounds. *World Journal of Surgery*, **7**, 641–645.

Marks, R. (1986) Assessment of wound dressings, in (eds) Turner, T.D., Schmidt, T.D., Harding, K.G., *Advances in Wound Management*. John Wiley & Sons, Chichester.

Meers, P.D. (1981) Report on the National Survey of Infection in Hospitals. *Journal of Hospital Infection*, **2** (8), 31–39.

Minns, J., Whittle, D. (1992) A simple photographic recording system for pressure sore assessment. *Journal of Tissue Viability*, **2** (4), 126.

Myers M.B., Cherry, G. (1984) Zinc and the healing of chronic leg ulcers. *American Journal of Surgery*, **120**, 77–81.

NHS Executive (1998) *Achieving Effective Practice*. Department of Health, London.

Plassmann, P. (1998) Wound measurement techniques, in (eds) Leaper, D., Cherry, G., Cockbill, S., Dealey, C., Flanagan, M., Hofman, D., *et al.*, *Proceedings of the EWMA/Journal of Wound Care Spring Conference*. Macmillan Magazines Ltd, London.

Plassmann, P., Jones, B.F., Ring, E.F.J. (1993) Assessment of a non-contact instrument to measure the volume of leg ulcers, in (eds) Harding, K.G., Cherry, G., Dealey, C., Turner, T.D., *Proceedings of the 2nd European Conference on Advances in Wound Management*. Macmillan Magazines Ltd, London.

Resch, C.S., Kerner, E., Robson, M.C., Heggers, J.P., Scherer, M., Boertman, J.A.,

Schileru, R. (1988) Pressure sore volume measurement, a technique to document and record wound healing. *Journal of American Geriatric Society*, **36**, 444–446.

van Riet Paap, E., Mekkes, J.R., Estevez, O., Westerhof, W. (1991) A new colour video image analysis system for the objective assessment of wound healing in secondary healing ulcers. *Wounds*, **3** (1), 41.

Rundgren, A., Nordehammar, A., Bjornestol, A., Magnusson, H., Nelson, C. (1990) Pressure sores in hospitalised geriatric patients. Background factors, treatment, long-term follow-up. *Care – Science and Practice*, **8** (3), 100–103.

Stewart, A.J., Leaper, D.J. (1987) Treatment of chronic leg ulcers in the community: a comparative trial of Scherisorb and Iodosorb. *Phlebology*, **2**, 115–121.

Thomas, S. (1990) *Wound Management and Dressings*. Pharmaceutical Press, London.

Thomas, S., Jones, M., Shutler, S., Andrews, A. (1996) All you need to know about maggots. *Nursing Times*, **92** (46), 63–76.

Thomas, S., Tucker, C.A. (1989) Sorbsan in the management of leg ulcers. *Pharmaceutical Journal*, **243**, 706–709.

Vowden, K. (1995) Common problems in wound care: wound and ulcer measurement. *British Journal of Nursing*, **4** (13), 775–779.

Wallace, P. (1994) *Polaroid Instant Record*. Wordpower Publishing, Welwyn.

Chapter 4
Wound Management Products

4.1 INTRODUCTION

There are many wound management products available and much conflicting advice on how they should be used. Many nurses have a great interest in this subject. They take a justifiable pride in the acquired skills which facilitate dressing change. Recent developments have demonstrated a need to change or adapt traditional practices.

Wound management products include topical agents as well as dressings. A topical agent is one which is applied to a wound. A dressing is a covering on a wound which is intended to promote healing and provide protection from further injury. The Department of Health (DOH) divides dressings into primary and secondary. A primary dressing is one which is used in direct contact with damaged tissue. A secondary dressing is superimposed over the primary dressing.

4.2 THE DEVELOPMENT OF DRESSINGS THROUGH THE AGES

In *L'Ingenue*, Voltaire (1767) described history as a 'tableau of crimes and misfortunes'. A study of the dressings used through the ages suggests that there may be some truth in this. Some of the treatments used on the wounded were bizarre, if not horrific, whilst others are still familiar today.

4.2.1 Early days

The earliest record of any dressing can be found on the Edwin Smith Papyrus. Edwin Smith was an American Egyptologist who bought the papyrus from a trader in Luxor in 1862. He was unable to translate it and its contents were unknown until a complete translation was published in 1930 (Zimmerman & Veith, 1961). The papyrus is dated at around 1700 BC, but it is a copy of original manuscripts which date back to around 3000–2500 BC. A variety of dressings are mentioned including grease, honey, lint and fresh meat, which was valued for its haemostatic properties. Adhesive strapping was made by applying gum to strips of linen (Forrest, 1982).

As the power of ancient Egypt waned, the Greek civilisation gradually developed. Amongst the men who made their mark at this time was Hippocrates (c. 460–377 BC) who laid the basis for scientific medicine with his emphasis on careful observation. For the most part, he considered that wounds should be kept clean and dry. He recommended tepid water, wine and vinegar for cleansing wounds. If a wound showed signs of inflammation, he suggested applying a cataplasm or poultice to the area around the wound to soften the tissues and to allow free drainage of pus (Zimmerman & Veith, 1961). He also used propolis, a hard resinous material produced by bees, to help in the healing of sores and ulcers (Trevelyn, 1997). Hippocrates gave the first definition of healing by first intention, where the skin edges are held in approximation to each other, and secondary intention where there is tissue loss and the skin edges are far apart.

Some of these concepts can also be found in the writings of Sushruta, an Indian surgeon who lived sometime between the sixth century BC and the sixth century AD. His surgical textbook the *Sushruta Samhita* has been used as a basis for later writers. Sushruta described 14 different types of dressings made from silk, linen, wool and cotton (Zimmerman & Veith, 1961). He also placed great emphasis on the importance of cleanliness. Meade (1968) describes Sushruta's recommendations for the management of wounds involving the intestines. First, black ants were applied and then the intestines were washed in milk and lubricated with clarified butter before they were returned to their normal position. He differed from Hippocrates on the matter of the most appropriate diet for patients. Sushruta considered meat, normally forbidden to Hindus, an important factor, whereas Hippocrates recommended the restriction of food and gave his patients only water to drink (Zimmerman & Veith, 1961).

During the Roman Empire oil and wine were commonly applied to wounds. Reference to this was made by the Gospel-writer St Luke in the parable of the Good Samaritan; Luke describes the Good Samaritan pouring oil and wine onto the wounds and then applying bandages.

Celsus compiled a history of the development of medicine from the time of Hippocrates to AD 100 with great detail of the practices of his time. Although it is believed that Celsus was not a physician, he was the first to give a definition of inflammation. He listed the cardinal signs as redness, heat, pain and swelling; he advocated the cleansing of wounds to remove foreign bodies before suturing and also expected wounds to suppurate, that is, to form pus (Meade, 1968). A Roman scholar, Pliny, described the use of propolis to soften induration and reduce swelling; he also noted that it healed sores when healing seemed impossible (Trevelyn, 1997).

It is, however, Galen who stands out as the person whose work has had lasting impact on wound management. Galen (AD 129–199) worked as the surgeon to the gladiators in Pergamun and later as physician to the Emperor Marcus Aurelius. He wrote many books, some of which survived him and were seen as the ultimate in medical knowledge for many centuries. He is particularly known for his theory of laudable pus ('*pus bonem et laudabile*') i.e. that the development of pus is necessary for healing and should, therefore, be actively promoted. Galen found the application of writing ink, cobwebs and Lemnian clay to wounds to be efficacious (Forrest, 1982). In reviewing his achievements, Duin and Sutcliffe (1992) considered that, although in some ways Galen considerably expanded medical knowledge, he also held it back for a thousand years.

After the fall of the Roman Empire, cultural influence moved eastwards and the Arab doctors of Islam further developed medical knowledge. However, their wound care was based on Galenic teaching. Various cleansing agents were used at this time. They included turpentine, lizard's dung and pigeon's blood. It is difficult to see the benefit of these substances today. Cooked honey and myrrh were used as astringents to reduce the amount of exudate produced by the wound.

In the Middle Ages the Church taught of the relationship between physical and spiritual health and also supplied most of the healthcare provision outside the home. This resulted in the Church having control over many aspects of medicine, such as giving support to Galenic teaching. Thus, the belief in the theory of laudable pus persisted and little advancement was made until the nineteenth century. But, there were a few glimmers in the darkness.

In the thirteenth century, the medical school at Salerno in Italy was regarded as the premier training school. One of the expert surgeons who graduated from Salerno was Hugo of Lucca. Although none of his writings have survived, they were cited by his famous pupil, Theodoric (1205–1296). Theodoric disagreed with the concept of laudable pus; he considered that it prolonged healing. Instead he advocated cleaning a wound with wine, debriding it and removing all foreign matter, suturing the wound edges and then applying a protective dressing. Unfortunately, his work was discredited and gradually his ideas disappeared until the twentieth century when his theories were again discovered in Italy (Popp, 1995).

Kirkpatrick and Naylor (1997) have described the contents of a surgical treatise dated 1446 and believed to be the work of Thomas Morstede (1380–1450) who was a London surgeon. The treatise provides detailed information about the classification of ulcers and their treatment. The step-by-step approach describes how to enlarge the mouth of the ulcer, then the processes of mortification (debridement), mundification (cleansing) and fleshing (encouragement of granulation tissue). The recipes for the various topical applications are provided for the reader. They include items such as sage leaves, wormwood, white Gascony wine, alum and honey for mundification. The recipe for a treatment for fleshing involved stirring the mixture for the length of time it took to say two creeds.

With the discovery of gunpowder, warfare changed. Gunshot wounds were believed to be poisonous. In order to treat them, surgeons began to undertake more amputation of limbs. The standard practice was to use boiling oil to cauterise the stump. Ambrose Paré (1510–1590) was a surgeon well versed in this practice. One day he did not have enough boiling oil and applied a mixture of egg yolks, oil of roses and turpentine instead. To his amazement his patients made better progress than usual. He then began to question the benefits of the traditional teaching of laudable pus.

However, Paré was still a man of his times. He spent two years trying to bribe another surgeon to reveal the recipe for a special balm made by boiling young puppies in oil of lilies, then adding earthworms prepared with turpentine of Venice.

Another surgeon worthy of mention is Heister (1683–1758). In his *General System of Surgery* he reviewed the range of dressings available, listing sticking plaster, compresses and bandages.

4.2.2 Nineteenth and early twentieth century developments

The Crimean War led to a huge demand for dressings. Various types of dressings were produced in the workhouses which were a source of cheap labour: charpie was made from unravelled cloth; oakum was old rope which had been unpicked and teased into fluff; tow was made from broken, ravelled flax fibres; lint is linen which has been scraped on one side. All of these dressings were washed and reused many times. They gradually became quite soft, but they were not very absorbent.

The credit for the first absorbent dressing must go to Gamgee (1828–1886). He found that cotton wool could be made absorbent by removing the oily matter within it. He then covered the cotton wool with bleached gauze to make dressing pads (Lawrence, 1987). Gamgee tissue is still available today.

During the course of World War I, more and more severely wounded soldiers had to wait several days to receive anything more than a simple field dressing. As a result, many wounds became infected and gangrenous. Antiseptics were developed to help resolve this problem. In particular, two similar antiseptic solutions came into use. They were Eusol (Edinburgh University Solution of Lime) and Dakin's solution. Other antiseptics such as iodine, carbolic acid, and mercury and aluminium chloride were also available.

Sinclair and Ryan (1993) have reviewed some of the medical literature of 1915 to identify thinking at that time on the use of antiseptics. Bond (1915) considered that it was important to apply a 'germicide' as early as possible to wounds which were almost certain to be infected. British soldiers were advised to carry tincture of iodine so that they could apply it immediately to any gunshot wounds (Mayo-Robson, 1915). However, Herzog (1915) writing of the German experience in the battle field reported that he had seen a number of soldiers suffering from dermatitis of the skin around the wound as a result of the indiscriminate use of iodine.

At this time, Lumière devised a dressing called *tulle gras*, a gauze impregnated with paraffin. Sphagnum moss was also used as it was found to be twice as absorbent as cotton wool. It could also be impregnated with antiseptics and sterilised. Eupad was a dressing designed for use on leg ulcers. It was a Eusol preparation made up with a mixture of boracic and bleach. Another popular type of dressing was Emplastrums. These were made of white leather spread with a plaster mass, to which some type of medication was often added (Turner, 1986).

During World War II an American neurosurgeon called Eldridge Campbell was with a field hospital in Italy. In 1943 there was a great deal of heavy fighting and many casualties. Some of the Italian doctors who were involved in caring for these patients proposed a method of wound care that involving cleansing and debriding the wound and then suturing it. This was contrary to current practice of the day which recommended packing with vaseline gauze and immobilisation. Campbell was impressed by this method of healing and eventually traced its origins back to the thirteenth century and Theodoric. In describing this fascinating piece of medical history, Popp (1995) concludes that it demonstrates the problems of entrenched views that are not questioned, such as the teachings of Galen, and the dangers of summarily dismissing new ideas.

4.2.3 The British pharmaceutical codices

The first *British Pharmaceutical Codex* was published in 1907. It provided information on all the drugs and medicinal preparations in common use throughout the British Empire. Turner (1986) has reviewed the dressings listed in the earliest British pharmaceutical codices and compared them with more recent lists of dressings in the *British Pharmacopoeia*. He found that the list from 1923 contains much that is familiar today. Table 4.1 compares the 1923 list with the 1980 list, showing that little has changed in the intervening years. Gauzes, cotton wool pads and bandages can be seen as very popular methods of wound care. Turner suggests that it is only in the last 20 years that any attempt has been made to design materials which are actually functional. Prior to that, dressings were made from materials that happened to come to hand.

Table 4.1 Comparison of surgical dressings 1923 and 1980.

1923		1980	
Gauzes, medicated and unmedicated	(13)	Gauze products	(11)
Cotton wools medicated and unmedicated	(15)	Cotton wool pads (eye)	(1)
Tows, medicated and unmedicated	(14)	Dressing pads	(2)
Lints, medicated and unmedicated	(8)	Impregnated gauze	(3)
Gauze and cotton tissues	(2)	Gauze and cotton tissues	(2)
Jaconet, oiled silk, etc.	(4)	Ribbon gauze	(3)
Bandages	(9)	Bandages	(15)
Emplastrums	(32)	Adhesive pads	(2)
		Foams	(3)
		Contact layers	(2)
		Absorbent cotton	(2)
		Medicated bandages	(4)

4.3 TRADITIONAL TECHNIQUES

These days nurses can expect to perform the vast majority of dressings, other than simple first-aid treatments applied in the home or work place. But this was not always the case: originally dressings were carried out by doctors; then medical students, particularly those on surgical wards, were trained to change dressings; by the 1930s, the task was given to experienced sisters, and ultimately, it became a recognised nursing task.

During the 1930s and 1940s, as the care of wounds gradually came into the nursing domain, much mystique became attached to the subject. This was exaggerated with the development of an aseptic, usually non-touch, dressing technique. Merchant (1988), when reviewing the literature on this subject, concluded that the procedure that was developed in the 1940s was still being used at the end of the 1980s, even though most hospitals had changed to a central sterile supply system by the early 1970s.

In the early days, large water sterilisers were used for preparing the equipment for an aseptic procedure; one was usually found on every ward. It was the task of the night nurses to boil all the metal bowls, receivers and gallipots, ready for the morning dressing round. The dressings were packed in drums and sent to a central point for sterilising. It was left to the ward sister to choose what went into the drum: commonly, gauze squares, cotton wool balls and wadding were used. In many hospitals nurses wore masks and gowns – a practice that has gradually disappeared. Usually two nurses carried out the dressing: a clean nurse and a dirty nurse. Much attention was paid to the position of the equipment on top of the trolley and to the frequency and timing of hand washing.

All wounds were re-dressed once or twice daily. The wound was thoroughly cleaned using cotton wool balls and forceps. The method of wiping across the wound surface varied from hospital to hospital. Figure 4.1 shows some of the common methods. The Hippocratic principle of keeping wounds clean and dry became adapted to 'allowing wounds to dry up'. Mostly gauze preparations were used, but gradually all sorts of dubious practices crept in. There have been reports of Marmite, eggs and even toast used on wounds (Dubranski, 1983; Johnson, 1987).

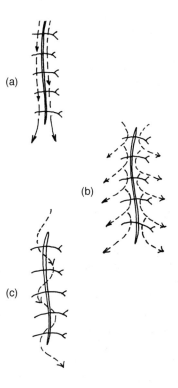

(a)

(b)

(c)

Fig. 4.1 Some of the common methods used for wound cleansing: (a) 'one wipe and away', swabbing along the length of the wound; (b) swabbing in short sweeps away from sutures; (c) rubbing along the length of the wound.

A wide variety of pharmaceutical preparations have also been applied without any recognition of the need for evidence-based care. Several studies have shown the extensive range of dressings being used in different areas. Murray (1988) found that within her health authority an amazing selection of pharmaceutical products were in use; 18 different cleansing agents, 53 substances left in contact with open wounds and 24 products used for packing wounds. Millward (1989) found 19 different substances being used on pressure sores within one hospital. Walsh and Ford (1989) have discussed the rituals in nursing, much of which can be applied to wound care. The common reasons for choosing a dressing could be listed as:

(1)   'We always do it that way here.'
(2)   'Sister said so.'
(3)   'I have used this dressing for the last 30 years, why should I change?'

Many nurses will have been trained to use these ritualistic methods. It is only recently that there has been a critical evaluation of these methods and changes made to a more evidence-based approach.

4.4 THE USE OF LOTIONS

A variety of lotions are used in wound care, primarily for wound cleansing. The aims of wound cleansing are to remove any foreign matter such as gravel or soil, to remove any loose surface debris such as necrotic tissue and to remove any remnants of the previous dressing. A study by Thomlinson (1987) considered the various ways that swabs could be wiped across the wound surface. The results showed that the action of cleansing did not reduce the number of bacteria on the wound surface, but simply redistributed them.

4.4.1 Antiseptics

After saline, the commonest type of lotion in use is an antiseptic. An antiseptic can be defined as a non-toxic disinfectant which can be applied to skin or living tissues and has the ability to destroy vegetative compounds, such as bacteria, by preventing their growth. If they are simply used to wipe across the wound surface they will have little effect. Antiseptics need to be in contact with bacteria for about 20 minutes before they actually destroy them (Russell *et al.*, 1982). In some instances they can be applied in the form of soaks or incorporated into dressings, ointments or creams.

However, research using experimental wounds in the animal model have demonstrated antiseptics have toxic effects which need to be weighed against any advantages obtained from their use. In the late 1980s and early 1990s there was considerable debate about the use of antiseptics. Much of it centred round the use of Eusol, but all types of antiseptics were included. At one point the United Kingdom Central Council (UKCC) received at least one enquiry a week about accountability and the use of Eusol (Pyne, personal communication). Many nurses felt that they were failing their patients if they complied with medical instruction to use it. Doctors were at first bewildered that nurses were questioning their practice and then became more intransigent. Stories were rife that nurses were being disciplined for refusing to use Eusol. Doctors were said to be taking nurses from one ward and placing them on another to make sure that patients got their Eusol dressing. Many papers and letters were written on the topic supporting one view or the other and the subject was hotly debated at conferences. An example is a series of letters published in the *British Medical Journal* during 1992 which ranged from calling for clinical trials (Leaper, 1992) to recriminations against nurses who were accused of being too naïve to see that they were being manipulated by the dressings' manufacturers (Coady, 1992).

After a while all the hype died away and the subject is now rarely discussed. A search in an electronic database revealed only one paper on Eusol in the last five years compared with 33 in the five years prior to that. Perhaps, as the level of evidence in respect of modern wound management products has increased, there is a greater willingness to put the role of antiseptics into perspective. Indiscriminate use of antiseptics is generally recognised as inappropriate. Healthcare professionals are increasingly aware that evidence is required to support the use of any antiseptic. It is no longer adequate for an individual to claim that anecdotal evidence of a 20-year period is all the evidence that is necessary. There is also a recognition that there may be a limited use for antiseptics in wound care. Each of the common antiseptics will be listed in turn and their advantages and disadvantages discussed.

Cetrimide

This is useful for its detergent properties – particularly for the initial cleansing of traumatic wounds or the removal of scabs and crusts in skin disease. It should not be used in contact with the eye. It is rapidly inactivated by organic material. Two dangers should be noted: it can cause skin irritation and sensitivity, and it is readily contaminated by bacteria, especially *Pseudomonas aeruginosa*. It is mostly only used in accident and emergency departments for initial cleansing of wounds rather than as a routine cleanser. It is available as a cream or as a lotion in combination with chlorhexidine. Morgan (1993) suggests that cetrimide should be used with caution in restricted circumstances rather than as a general cleanser.

Chlorhexidine

Chlorhexidine is used in a variety of aqueous formulations. It is effective against Gram-positive and Gram-negative organisms. Brennan *et al.* (1986) found that it has a low toxicity to living cells. Tatnall *et al.* (1990) undertook a similar study to identify the toxicity of several antiseptics when used on cultured keratinocytes (used for grafts). They found chlorhexidine to be the least toxic, but considered that antiseptics should not be used over these graft sites. Kearney *et al.* (1988) found that it could maintain its antimicrobial levels for a period of time when impregnated into a dressing. However, the efficacy of chlorhexidine is rapidly diminished in the presence of organic material such as pus or blood (Reynolds, 1982). Chlorhexidine is sometimes combined with cetrimide. Chlorhexidine seems to have little part to play in general wound care.

Hydrogen peroxide 3% (10 vols)

This has an oxidising effect which destroys anaerobic bacteria. However, it loses its effect when it comes in contact with organic material such as pus or cotton gauze.

The oxidising effect is also beneficial in removing slough from wounds. A study by Graber *et al.* (1975) found that hydrogen peroxide assisted in the rapid removal of slough, but, if it was used on a granulating wound, air blisters formed which burst and led to further breakdown of the wound.

Lineaweaver *et al.* (1985) showed that hydrogen peroxide was cytotoxic to fibroblasts unless diluted to a strength of 0.003%. This dilution is not effective against bacteria. O'Toole *et al.* (1996) found that even in concentrations 1000-fold less than 3% dilution it inhibits keratinocyte migration and proliferation. There is also a report of an incident where an air embolism occurred after irrigation with hydrogen peroxide (Sleigh & Linter, 1985). The use of hydrogen peroxide should be restricted to very sloughy wounds and it should never be used in cavity wounds. Some would also recommend limiting the number of applications or irrigating the wound with saline after use.

Hydrogen peroxide is also available in a stabilised form as a 1.5% cream. In this form the antiseptic action is prolonged.

Iodine

Iodine is a broad-spectrum antiseptic and is available in both an alcohol and an aqueous solution. The aqueous solution is used in wound care, usually as povidone-iodine 10% which contains 1% available iodine. It is used as a skin disinfectant and to clean grossly infected wounds. McLure and Gordon (1992) found it to be effective against methicillin-resistant *Staphylococcus aureus*. Several studies have questioned the value of using povidone-iodine. It is cytotoxic to fibroblasts unless diluted to 0.001%, retards epithelialisation and lowers the tensile strength of the wound (Lineaweaver *et al.*, 1985). Brennan and Leaper (1985) found that povidone-iodine 5% damaged the microcirculation of the healing wound, but a 1% solution was innocuous. Becker (1986) reported that when operating on contaminated head and neck cases he irrigated 18 with povidone-iodine and 17 with isotonic saline. Some 28% of wounds became infected, all of which had been irrigated with povidone-iodine.

Povidone-iodine is also available in ointment, spray and powder form and impregnated into dressings.

Iodine should not be used for patients with thyroid disease or who have a sensitivity to the product.

Although iodine was one of the antiseptics that fell from favour at the beginning of the 1990s, it seems to be making something of a comeback. Gilchrist (1997) reported on the conclusions of a consensus meeting to discuss the role of iodine in wound care. The group comprised clinicians, scientists and representatives of industry and met under the auspices of the European Tissue Repair Society. After debating all the literature they concluded that there may be a role for iodine in the acute management of surgically drained abscesses and in clinically infected chronic wounds. Further research is still required to clarify the best formulation of iodine and how it can most effectively be used.

Potassium permanganate 0.01%

This is mostly used on heavily exuding eczematous conditions, mostly associated with leg ulceration. It is mildly deodorising and has slight disinfectant properties. It has been found to cause staining of the skin.

It is most easily used in the form of tablets. One tablet dissolved in four litres of water provides a 0.01% solution.

Proflavine

This has a mild bacteriostatic effect on Gram-positive organisms, but not on Gram-negative bacteria. There has been little research to demonstrate its value. Although it is available as a lotion it is mostly used as an aqueous cream. However, the proflavine is not released from the cream into the wound, so has no effect on the bacteria.

Silver nitrate 0.5%

Silver nitrate is rarely used as a lotion. It stains the skin black, and prolonged use causes hyponatraemia, hypokalaemia and hypocalcaemia. It is not recommended.

Sodium hypochlorite

This comes in several forms, the commonest being Eusol, Dakin's solution and Milton. It was originally used on heavily infected wounds during World War I. Dakin suggested that for it to be effective, it should be used in large volumes (Thomas, 1990).

Several research studies have been undertaken which suggest that the hypochlorite salts may have little beneficial effect and do much harm. Bloomfield *et al.* (1985) found that they cause irritation to both the wound and the surrounding skin; have a cumulative effect causing redness, pain and oedema; and prolong the inflammatory stage of healing. Sodium hypochlorite is cytotoxic to fibroblasts, unless diluted to a strength of 0.0005%, and retards epithelialisation (Lineaweaver *et al.*, 1985). Brennan and Leaper (1985) found that it caused considerable damage to the microcirculation of the wound. The antiseptic effect is lost when it comes in contact with organic material such as pus or gauze. A study describing the use of Eusol and liquid paraffin on leg ulcers was undertaken by Daltrey and Cunliffe (1981). They found no significant evidence of antibacterial activity. Thomas (1986) found that about 100 ml of Milton were required to dissolve 1 g of yellow slough. He further calculated that, using ribbon gauze 2.5 cm $\times$ 1 m soaked in 5 ml of hypochlorite solution, about 100 dressing changes would be required to remove 5 g of slough (Thomas, 1990).

Humzah *et al.* (1996) surveyed 124 plastic surgeons in the UK regarding their views on the use of Eusol. They had responses from 95 (77%) of the surgeons. Analysis of the responses found that 82% still used Eusol when it was available and the majority (88%) used it for sloughy wounds. The authors state that Eusol should only be used on dirty, sloughy wounds for a short period and never in clean wounds (i.e. granulating wounds). They go on to state that in view of the lack of controlled evidence against Eusol there needs to be an effective clinical trial. However, as Eusol is virtually banned in many places they suggest it may be too late.

It is also interesting to consider that where alternative modern products have replaced Eusol, it has not been missed at all. Humzah et al. (1996) also recognise that the plastic surgeons employed other methods as well for desloughing wounds. Overall, Eusol is an outmoded product whose disadvantages far outweigh any slight advantage there may be in its use.

4.4.2 Antibiotics

A range of antibiotics is available in topical form. They are potentially hazardous and they are not always absorbed into the wound. There is considerable risk of sensitisation to the patient as well as the development of resistant organisms. Systemic antibiotics are the treatment of choice when treating infected wounds because the infection may be too deep for topical antibiotics to penetrate.

D'Arcy (1972) recommends that any antibiotic that is used systemically should not be applied to the skin. However, antibiotics that are not appropriate for systemic use may be developed for use on the skin or in wound care. This means that creams, gels, ointments or impregnated dressings containing gentamicin, tetracycline, fusidic acid or chlortetracycline hydrochloride should not be used, as these antibiotics are used systemically. Neomycin is no longer used systemically, but topical use may cause systemic side-effects such as ototoxicity. One preparation which would seem to be of benefit in wound care is mupirocin.

Mupirocin is used predominantly for treating methicillin-resistant *Staphylococcus aureus* (MRSA) either in skin infections or in nasal colonisation. Several studies have demonstrated its efficacy in treating MRSA in burn wounds (Rode et al., 1989; Deng et al., 1995, Trilla & Miro, 1995). However, Cookson (1998) warns of the potential dangers of resistant bacteria. He cites a number of reported cases of mupirocin-resistant bacteria to support his arguments. He proposes that prolonged and widespread use of mupirocin should be stopped, and a more judicious approach to its usage be adopted.

4.4.3 Saline 0.9%

This is the only completely safe cleansing agent and is the treatment of choice for use on most wounds. Manufacturers recommend it is used in conjunction with many of the modern wound management products. Saline is presented in sachets, small plastic containers that allow the saline to be squirted on to the wound and also in aerosols. These last two presentations are more widely used in the community.

4.4.4 Tap water

Tap water is being used more frequently on a variety of wounds. In particular, on areas already colonised such as wounds following rectal surgery or leg ulcers. Many patients may bath or shower prior to dressing change. There seems to be little point in then 'cleansing' the wound. However, the bath or shower should be thoroughly cleaned afterwards to avoid cross-infection. Hall-Angeras (1992) randomly allocated 617 patients with trauma wounds to either sterile saline or lukewarm tap water for wound cleansing. A significantly higher number of wounds cleansed with saline were infected compared with the tap water group. The authors suggest that this might be because of the profuse rinsing that could be achieved with tap water.

4.5 CLINICALLY EFFECTIVE WOUND MANAGEMENT PRODUCTS

Originally dressings were seen merely as coverings which could provide some protection to the wound. The products currently available are much more sophisticated. There are so many products to choose from that it can cause considerable confusion. There is no single perfect dressing but an 'identikit' list of criteria can be established. The requirements of a specific wound may not need all of the criteria listed. Selection can be assisted if the nurse has:

- assessed the wound and identified the specific objectives for the wound at that time;
- an understanding of what can be reasonably expected from a dressing;
- access to information regarding the characteristics and effectiveness of the range of dressings available to the nurse.

The characteristics of a clinically effective wound management product will be considered below. Dressings are generally considered in relation to their performance and their handling qualities. Performance relates to their ability to promote healing.

4.5.1 Providing an effective environment

The qualities which will promote an effective environment for healing are:

(1) Maintaining a moist environment.
(2) Antibacterial properties.
(3) Fluid-handling properties.

(1) Maintaining a moist environment
The importance of a moist environment was identified by the work of George Winter (1962). His research has had a profound effect on wound management. He compared the effect of leaving superficial wounds exposed to form a scab with the effect of applying a vapour permeable film dressing, using an animal model. Epithelialisation was twice as fast in those wounds covered with a film dressing. This was because the dressing maintains humidity on the wound surface. Thus, the epithelial cells were able to slide across the surface of the wound; whereas in the exposed wounds the epithelial cells had to burrow beneath the scab, beneath the dried exudate and beneath the dessicated layers of cells to find a moist layer to allow movement across the wound.

Later studies have confirmed this finding and identified other benefits as well. May (1984), Eaglstein, (1985) and Alvarez and Dellanoy (1987) all found local wound pain was considerably reduced in a moist environment, possibly because the nerve endings did not dry out. Studies by Freidman and Su (1983), and Kaufman and Hirshowitz (1983), showed that the moist environment enhanced natural autolytic processes, breaking down necrotic tissue.

(2) Antibacterial properties
All dressings should have some degree of antibacterial properties. Some will have constituents which are bactericidal and others provide a barrier between the wound and the environment. The benefits of the dressing as a barrier are two-fold. It prevents contamination of the wound by stopping airborne micro-organisms penetrating through to the wound. Also, bacteria on the wound surface are prevented from escaping into the environment and causing cross infection. However, a soaked or leaking dressing provides a pathway for bacteria in both directions.

(3) Fluid-handling properties
Although the wound surface should remain moist, excessive moisture causes maceration of the surrounding skin. The precise balance that needs to be maintained by the dressing between moisture and absorbency is still not certain.

4.5.2 The handling qualities of an effective wound management product

These qualities can be listed as:

(1) Easy to apply.
(2) Conformability.
(3) Easy to remove.
(4) Comfortable to 'wear'.
(5) Does not require frequent dressing change.

(1) Easy to apply
A major advantage of many of the modern products is that they are very simple and quick to apply. Realistically, this has helped to promote their use with the nurses who regularly provide wound care.

(2) Conformability
A dressing which conforms well to the shape of the wound is likely to assist in maintaining a moist environment and also provide an effective barrier for bacteria.

(3) Easy to remove
If a dressing is easy to remove it is less likely to damage any of the newly formed tissue in the wound; it is also less likely to be painful for the patient.

(4) Comfortable to 'wear'
Another advantage of many modern products is that they are comfortable for the patient when they are in situ. This means that the patient is more likely to want to comply with the treatment regime. In any case, there is no need for patients to suffer unnecessary pain or discomfort.

(5) Does not require frequent dressing change

The majority of modern products can be left in place for several days, depending on the wound and, particularly, the amount of exudate. This not only saves nursing time and reduces costs but also reduces the amount of interference with the wound. Reduction in the frequency of dressing change helps to reduce the opportunities for a drop in temperature on the wound surface. This can potentially occur at each dressing change. Myers (1982) studied 420 patients and found that, after wound cleansing, it was 40 minutes before the wound regained its original temperature. Furthermore, he found that it took three hours for mitotic activity to return to its normal rate. Patients also find less frequent dressing changes beneficial. Some patients find dressing change an ordeal and others, especially community patients, an inconvenience which disrupts their life.

4.5.3 Conclusions

It should be recognised that no one dressing provides the optimum environment for the healing of all wounds. Equally, it may be necessary to use more than one type of dressing during the healing of a wound. Many dressings will fulfil some of the criteria and they should be selected following careful assessment of the wound (see Chapter 3).

4.6 MODERN WOUND MANAGEMENT PRODUCTS

In order to make sense of all the dressings that are available, they can be divided into different categories. They can also be considered in terms of their suitability as a primary or secondary dressing on open wounds.

In the UK, not all the dressings are freely available in chemists' shops and pharmacies. Government restrictions control which dressings may be prescribed. This may considerably affect continuity and quality of care between hospital and community.

This section aims to describe the different categories of wound management products and some proprietary examples will be mentioned.

4.6.1 Absorbent pads

There are many versions of this type of dressing. Most are in the form of an absorbent core which is covered by a sleeve of gauze or synthetic material. These dressings are not suitable as a primary dressing on open wounds, but make an excellent secondary dressing, particularly when there is a heavy exudate.

4.6.2 Adhesive island dressings

These dressings consist of a central pad which is covered with a wider band of adhesive backing. They are lightweight and usually remain in position satisfactorily. There is little absorbent capacity in these dressings. They are widely used on postsurgical wounds which are healing by first intention, but are not suitable as a primary dressing for open wounds.

4.6.3 Alginates

Alginate dressings contain calcium or sodium alginate which is derived from seaweed. There are several types of alginate including Algosteril®, Kaltogel®, Kaltostat®, Comfeel®, SeaSorb®, Sorbsan® and Tegagen®. This type of dressing is interactive because as it reacts with the wound its structure alters. As the dressing absorbs exudate it changes from a fibrous structure to a gel. These dressings are available in a variety of formats – flat dressings, rope or ribbon, extra absorbent versions and with an adhesive backing. They are appropriate for moderate or heavily exuding wounds and may require a secondary dressing. They should not be used on wounds with no or low exudate.

4.6.4 Antibacterials

The products in this category are quite different. Arglaes® controlled release is a film dressing with a polymer containing silver ions. It is effective against a range of bacteria including MRSA. Flamazine® is a cream containing silver sulphadiazine. It is effective against *Pseudomonas* and *Staphylococcus aureus*. It is widely used on burns. Metrotop® is a gel containing metronidazole. It reduces odour and anaerobic bacteria and is used on fungating tumours.

4.6.5 Antibiotics

See Section 4.4.2.

4.6.6 Antiseptics

See Section 4.4.1.

4.6.7 Beads

These dressings are sometimes referred to as dextranomers or xerogels. They are interactive dressings. There are several types available: Debrisan®, Iodoflex® and Iodosorb®. They consist of powder or beads which swell and gel in the presence of exudate. Various formats have developed because of the difficulties of application on to relatively shallow wounds. The beads have been incorporated into paste. The powder is also available as an ointment or as a slab of ointment. Iodoflex® and Iodosorb® also contain iodine, which is effective against a range of bacteria. These products should only be used on moderate to heavily exuding sloughy, necrotic or infected wounds. A secondary dressing is necessary.

4.6.8 Charcoal dressings

These dressings are made from activated charcoal cloth which has been found to be effective in absorbing the chemicals released from malodorous wounds. Infected, necrotic or fungating wounds may have a very unpleasant odour. The dressings come in two types, a charcoal pad, such as Actisorb Plus®, or a combination of dressing and charcoal such as Carbonet®, CliniSorb® or Lyofoam C®. The charcoal pad may be used in combination with other dressings. The combination dressing may need a secondary dressing.

4.6.9 Foams

Foam dressings may be made from polyurethane or silicone. They are available either as a flat foam dressing, such as Allevyn®, Lyofoam Extra® or Tielle® or as a filler for cavity wounds, such as Allevyn® cavity wound dressing or Cavi-Care®. These dressings come in a variety of presentations: flat foam, adhesive foam and tracheostomy dressings. Allevyn® cavity wound is a pre-formed foam stent which comes in two shapes and two sizes in each. Cavi-Care® is also a foam stent, but it has to be mixed with a catalyst and poured into the cavity where it takes up the shape of the wound. Foam dressings are best used on granulating or epithelialising wounds with some exudate.

4.6.10 Hydrocolloids

Hydrocolloids are a development from stoma products. They are interactive dressings consisting of a hydrocolloid base made from cellulose, gelatines and pectins and a backing made from a polyurethane film or foam. The technology has progressed since the original hydrocolloid dressings were introduced and a second generation of products are now available which have greater absorbency and hold exudate more effectively within the dressing. Examples of hydrocolloid dressings include: Comfeel® Plus, Cutinova Hydro®, Granuflex® (known as Duoderm® outside UK) and Tegasorb®. Several come in a wide range of sizes and variations such as a thinner than the standard dressing. No secondary dressing is necessary. Cutinova Hydro® has a greater absorptive capacity than other hydrocolloids as does Aquacel® a flat sheet dressing made from hydrocolloid fibres. Combiderm® is another variation of hydrocolloid technology. It is composed with several layers including a thin hydrocolloid and an island pad containing polyacrylate granules which hold the exudate within the pad. There are also two presentations for cavity wounds Aquacel Ribbon® and Cutinova Cavity®. Aquacel Ribbon® is a non-woven ribbon made from hydrocolloid fibres which gel as they absorb exudate. Cutinova Cavity® is a flat sheet which can be folded or cut into a ribbon shape. Initially it should only fill half the cavity because it swells as it absorbs exudate and moulds to the shape of the cavity. Hydrocolloids can be used on a wide range of wounds, but are most effective on the moderate-to-low exuding wounds. The two versions for cavity wounds have greater absorbency and are suitable for heavy-to-moderate exuding cavities.

4.6.11 Hydrogels

These dressings are made from insoluble polymers and have a large water content. The amorphous gels, such as GranuGel®, Intrasite® Gel, Nu-Gel® or Sterigel® may be used on a wide variety of wounds. They have the ability either to absorb exudate or to hydrate dry wounds such as necrotic eschar, thus encouraging debridement. They can be used on wounds with moderate to low exudate and in small cavities. The gel sheets such as 2nd Skin® or Vigilon® are best used on granulating moderate-to-low exuding wounds. They all require a secondary dressing.

4.6.12 Low adherent dressings

These types of dressing are low adherent rather than non-adherent. They have little if any absorbent capacity and are best on wounds with little exudate. They may be used to 'carry' a dressing such as an amorphous hydrogel; and mostly need to be used in combination with an absorbent pad. They do not provide a moist wound environment. Examples of this type of dressing are Melolin®, NA-Ultra®, Release®, Telfa® and Tricotex®.

4.6.13 Low adherent dressings (medicated)

Inadine® is a low adherent dressing which is impregnated with water-soluble povidone-iodine. It is suitable for moderate-to-low exuding infected wounds or for prophylaxis in minor traumatic wounds.

4.6.14 Paste bandages

These are cotton bandages impregnated with medicated paste. They are widely used on leg ulcers, particularly when the surrounding skin is eczematous or inflamed. Although they are an effective form of treatment, many patients develop allergies to the contents of the paste. It is wise to patch test the patient before applying a bandage. There are several types of bandage with different pastes such as zinc paste with ichthammol or zinc paste with calamine. A secondary bandage is required.

4.6.15 Streptokinase/streptodornase

This is an enzymatic preparation which is presented in the form of powder in a vial. It is reconstituted with normal saline to form a liquid or with a small amount of saline and a lubricating gel to form a jelly. Its action is to debride wounds and it is particularly useful on necrotic eschar. A semi-permeable film or gauze may be used as a secondary dressing. Varidase® is the only one of this type of dressing available in the UK. Recently there has been some debate about the use of streptokinase in wound care. Streptokinase is the thrombolytic agent of choice when treating acute myocardial infarction. It is given intravenously. However, following treatment, an immune response produces antibodies within five days which render further treatment ineffective for a period of up to six months. Some patients may have a reaction if given streptokinase in this period, which can range from mild hypersensitivity to anaphylactic shock. Bux et al. (1997) found the use of streptokinase/streptodornase on sloughy wounds caused an antibody reaction within a month which lasted up to six months. Healthcare professionals should be aware of this problem and avoid the use of this product on patients at risk of or who have recently suffered from myocardial infarction.

4.6.16 Tulles (non-medicated)

Tulles are also called paraffin gauze, which was originally known as *tulle gras*. It is made of open weave cotton or rayon impregnated with soft paraffin. Although the paraffin makes the dressing less adherent, it readily becomes incorporated into granulation tissue. A pattern can be seen on the wound surface when it is removed. It does not maintain a moist wound environment and has no absorbent capacity. It is widely used on minor burns and traumatic injuries. Examples are Jelonet®, Para-net®, Paratulle® and Unitulle®. Mepitel® has a similar structure but contains silicone gel rather than paraffin and does not cause the problems seen with paraffin gauze. A secondary dressing is required with these dressings.

4.6.17 Tulles (medicated)

Some types of tulles are impregnated with either antiseptics or antibiotics. The commonest type of antiseptic is chlorhexidine and it is present in Bactigras®, Chlorhexitulle® and Serotulle®. Inadine® is slightly different in that it is made of rayon. This dressing is impregnated with povidone-iodine ointment. These dressings are useful for superficial infected wounds. Two tulles are impregnated with antibiotics (Fucidin Intertulle® and Sofra-Tulle®). The use of these dressings is not recommended because of the problems of sensitivity and resistance of bacteria.

4.6.18 Vapour-permeable films

There is a wide range of these film dressings available. They provide a moist healing environment but have no absorbency, and should not be used on infected wounds. The method of application varies according to make. Most require a certain amount of skill and practice in application. Examples include Bioclusive®, Cutifilm®, Opsite® and Tegaderm®.

4.6.19 Vapour-permeable membranes

An advance on the film dressings are vapour-permeable products which have a certain amount of absorbency or exudate handling properties. Spyrosorb® and FlexiPore® are examples of this type of product. They have differing constructions. Products such as Omiderm®, Surfasoft® or Tegapore® allow exudate to pass through the dressing and can be left in place for several weeks whilst the outer dressings are changed.

4.7 NEW TECHNOLOGIES

As with any other aspect of healthcare, new developments in wound care are regularly announced. Sometimes they are variations on an older form of treatment and sometimes they are unique concepts. This section seeks to identify these innovations and consider the evidence to support their use.

4.7.1 Growth factors

Growth factors have been used for some time in wound care, although their use is still limited and they are not readily available. In the USA growth factors have primarily been used in wound care centres which utilise a comprehensive programme of full assessment and planned care. Many of the patients treated in these centres have leg or foot ulcers such as demonstrated in a randomised controlled trial undertaken by Knighton *et al.* (1990). They found a significantly higher rate of healing in those treated with growth factor solution compared with a blinded placebo.

In a debate on the use of growth factors, Arnold (1996) suggested that they have been shown in experimental studies to be more effective in improving defective healing than in accelerating normal healing. However, he considered that there was less clear evidence in studies of chronic wounds. Another issue is that growth factors are very expensive, which can raise any number of ethical dilemmas when only limited funds are available for providing patient care. Spencer *et al.* (1996) suggest that, although the results of clinical trials have so far been disappointing, the interest in the use of growth factors has led to a greater understanding of the physiological composition of different types of chronic wound.

4.7.2 Hyperbaric oxygen

Hyperbaric oxygen chambers have been used for many years for recompression therapy for divers with the bends or decompression illness. More recently they have also been used for non-healing wounds. Hyperbaric oxygen treatment has been defined as 'the patient breathing in 100% oxygen intermittently at a point higher than sea level pressure' (British Medical Association Board of Science and Education, 1993). The treatment is given by placing a patient inside a pressure chamber, which may be designed for one or more people. The length of treatments vary according to the condition being treated.

Hyperbaric oxygen has been used for a number of different wound types and has been shown to give mixed results. Brannen *et al.* (1997) randomised 125 burn patients to hyperbaric oxygen treatment or no treatment, all receiving standardised wound care. They found no statistical difference between the two groups and considered that they could find no benefit in its use. Neovius *et al.* (1997) compared 15 consecutive patients who had wound complications after surgery to the irradiated head and neck with 15 patients from a previous study. They found a significantly improved healing rate in the hyperbaric oxygen group compared with the control. Pizzorno *et al.* (1997) used hyperbaric oxygen therapy for 11 patients with Fournier's disease and considered that it was an effective adjunct treatment for this condition. Two studies looking at the use of this therapy for diabetic foot ulcers came to conflicting conclusions. Zamboni *et al.* (1997) compared five patients who refused hyperbaric oxygen treatment with five who had treatment and found a significantly reduced wound size in the treatment group compared with the control group. They advocated a large randomised controlled trial to evaluate definitively the effectiveness of hyperbaric oxygen for the diabetic foot. In contrast, Ciaravino *et al.* (1996) carried out a retrospective study of 54 patients with non-healing lower extremity wounds who had been treated with hyperbaric oxygen. They considered the results to be dismal with no wounds healing and only 11% showing any improvement. The average cost for the treatments was $14,000. The authors of this study concluded that it was difficult to justify using such an expensive, ineffective and complication-prone treatment.

It is obvious that the case for the use of hyperbaric oxygen is inconclusive. However, for most nurses the argument is academic as they are not likely to have access to such equipment.

4.7.3 Biosurgery

Biosurgery is another name for maggot or larvae therapy. The use, often inadvertent, of maggots in wounds has been recognised for centuries. Morgan (1995) chronicled the use of maggots from Mayan Indians through to the 1930s. He considered that the use of maggots fell into disrepute with the advent of antibiotics and aseptic wound care. He also noted the aesthetic problems with their usage. However, the use of larvae therapy is enjoying a resurgence of popularity at present.

Thomas *et al.* (1996) suggest this return in popularity might be in part because of the problems caused by resistant bacteria such as MRSA. They have developed a dedicated biosurgery unit which produces sterile larvae which can be sent anywhere in the UK. They arrive in a sealed container ready for use. The surrounding skin has to be protected with a hydrocolloid dressing. The larvae are inserted into a wound and kept in place with a net dressing sealed to the hydrocolloid surround. An absorbent pad provides an outer covering. Larvae should only be used in necrotic or sloughy wounds for debridement. Informed consent should be obtained from the patient before use of this treatment.

Although there has been much interest in larvae therapy, possibly because of the feelings of revulsion that it engenders, as yet there is little evidence to support its use. Most of the evidence is in the form of case studies, e.g. Thomas *et al.* (1996) and Jones and Thomas (1997). Church (1996) discussed the potential for this form of treatment, especially because of its relatively low cost, but also emphasised the need for rigorous scientific scrutiny.

4.7.4 Vacuum-assisted closure

Vacuum-assisted closure or VAC therapy is a device which applies a universal negative pressure to a wound encouraging blood flow and faster granulation (Baxandall, 1996). It comprises a foam sponge to fit into the wound, tubing to connect the foam to the pump via a canister to collect exudate (see Plate 14). The sponge is covered with a film dressing to create an air-tight seal. Pressure can be applied continuously or intermittently.

Vacuum-assisted closure was pioneered by Argenta and Morykwas in the USA.

They described the outcomes of 300 cases they have treated (Argenta and Mory-kwas, 1997); these wounds ranged from chronic to subacute, and acute wounds. They found it to be successful in 296 cases. Blackburn *et al.* (1998) reported using VAC therapy prior to skin grafting of large complex open wounds and found that they were able to get a minimum of a 95% take. Use of VAC has been reported by a number of plastic surgery centres (Russ *et al.*, 1997; Teot *et al.*, 1997; Voinchet *et al.*, 1997). Voinchet *et al.* (1997) warn that although VAC produces good quality healing it does have drawbacks. It reduces mobility in non-bedfast patients. It can be difficult to seal the wound when it is situated in awkward areas and it is very expensive. It has also not been subject to any comparative studies which would help to clarify its role in the management of complex wounds.

4.7.5 Tissue culture

Tissue culture describes the process whereby a small full-thickness section of skin is harvested from a patient or donor and then cultured in the laboratory to form large sheets of cells (cultured keratinocytes). The sheets of cells are then grafted on to a granulating wound completely free of any necrotic material. Autologous tissue (that taken from the patient) has been found to be more effective than allogeneic tissue (that taken from a donor); however, it can take more than a month to prepare (Kakibuchi *et al.*, 1996). Tissue culture has become well established since the early 1980s when the first clinical reports of its use appeared. More recent research has concentrated on improving the effectiveness of the product.

Wright *et al.* (1998) describe the use of a polyurethane foam dressing as a carrier for cultured keratinocytes. They found it was a useful vehicle, but that there was slow proliferation of cells. They suggest that cells should be expanded using the standard methods and then seeded on to the dressing. Myers *et al.* (1997) tested a hyaluronic membrane delivery system for cultured keratinocytes on an animal model and found that it gave a superior keratinocyte take. The researchers suggest that this system requires further investigation and clinical evaluation.

Kumagai *et al.* (1997) followed up 38 patients who had received autologous cultured keratinocyte grafts for over two years. They concluded that cultured tissue has a site specificity even after grafting and therefore, where it is possible, the maxim 'closer is best', which is applied to conventional skin grafting, should also be used for tissue cultures.

On the whole, cultured keratinocytes have been used by plastic surgeons parti-cularly for treating burn patients. However, they have also been used for treating leg ulcers that have not responded to other forms of treatment. In reviewing this, Kakibuchi *et al.* (1996) consider that it has not been an unqualified success as grafts have only shown a 10–20% take. Tissue culture is an important therapy for burn patients. It may have potential for a wider use, but needs some further development.

4.7.6 Tissue engineering

Tissue engineering takes tissue culture a step forward. It uses human dermal fibroblasts and cultures them on a biosynthetic scaffold. The fibroblasts proliferate

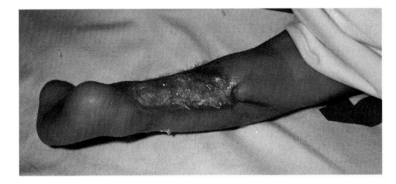

Plate 1 Contractures developing on a leg wound in an infant.

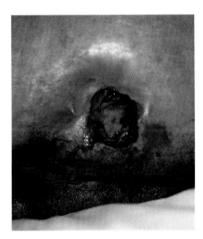

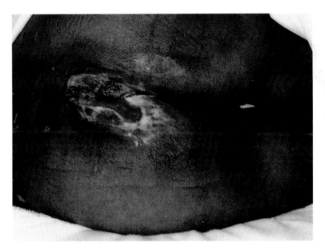

Plate 2 (above) An illustration of skin maceration from a heavily exuding wound.
Plate 3 (above right) A necrotic wound.
Plate 4 (below right) An infected wound.
Plate 5 (right) A sloughy wound.

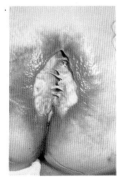

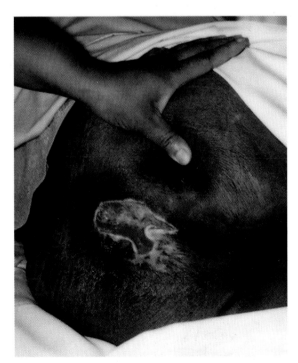

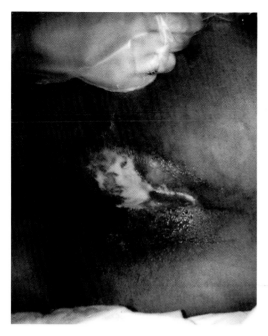

Plate 6 A granulating wound.

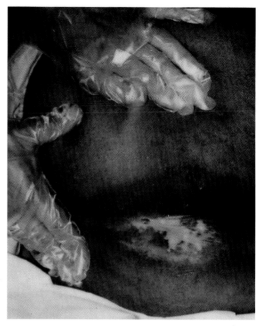

Plate 7 An epithelialising wound.

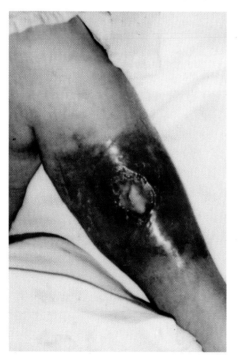

Plate 8 Contact dermatitis.

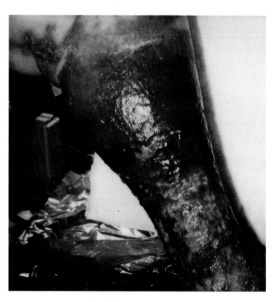

Plate 9 Irritant dermatitis.

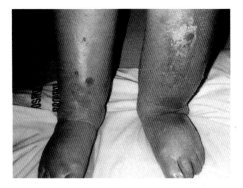

Plate 10 Oedematous legs with fragile skin and ulcers.

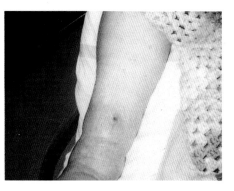

Plate 11 The same, one week later.

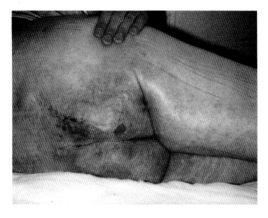

Plate 12 A patient with allergies to several dressings.

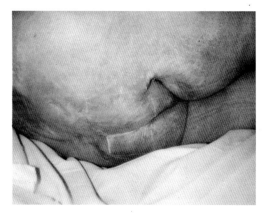

Plate 13 The same, after application of a protective skin wipe.

Plate 14 (left) VAC therapy equipment. Reproduced with kind permission of KCI Medical UK Ltd.

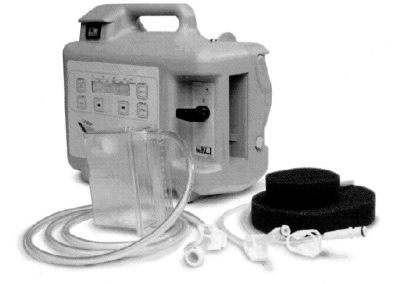

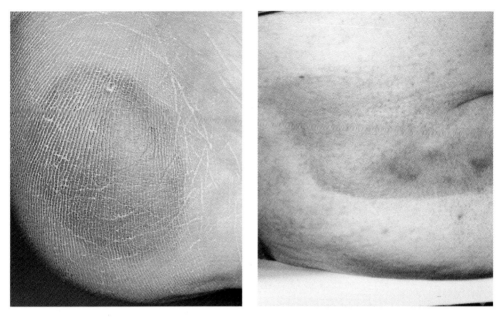

Plates 15 and 16 Non blanchable erythema of intact skin. This may be difficult to identify in darkly pigmented skins.

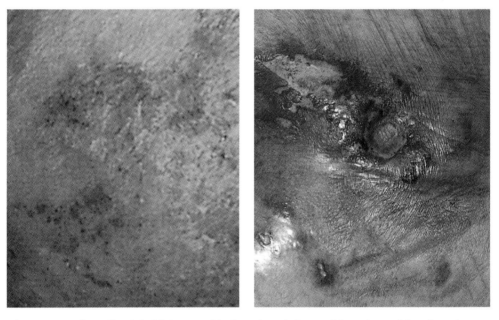

Plates 17 and 18 Partial thickness skin loss involving epidermis and/or dermis. The pressure sore is superficial and presents clinically as an abrasion, blister or shallow crater.

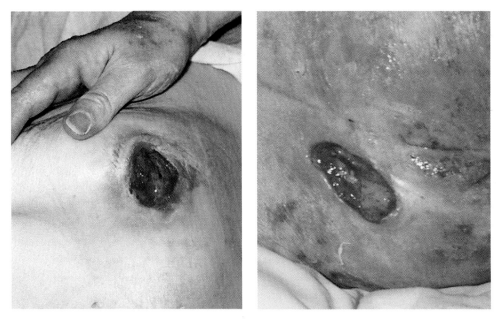

Plates 19 and 20 Full thickness skin loss involving damage or necrosis of subcutaneous tissue that may extend down to, but not through, underlying fascia. The pressure sore presents clinically as a deep crater with or without undermining of adjacent tissue.

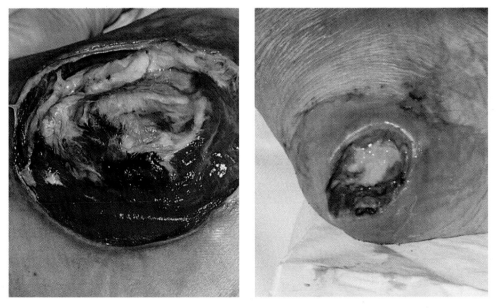

Plates 21 and 22 Full thickness skin loss with extensive destruction, tissue necrosis or damage to muscle, bone or supporting structures, e.g. tendon or joint capsule. Undermining and sinus tracts may also be associated with stage 4 pressure sores.
[Plates 15–22 Reproduced with permission of Huntleigh Healthcare Ltd.]

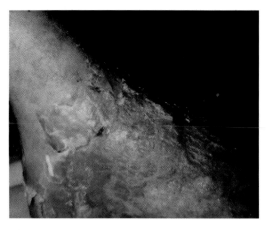

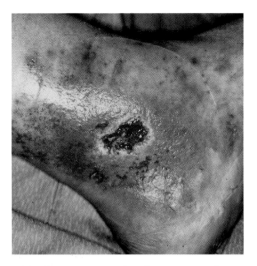

Plate 24 The management of skin scales.

Plate 23 An example of a venous ulcer.

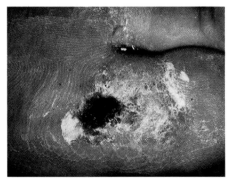

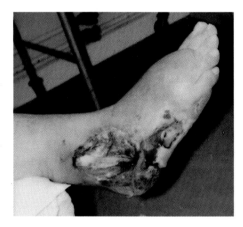

Plate 25a An arterial ulcer.

Plate 25b Advanced arterial ulcer: leg requires amputation.

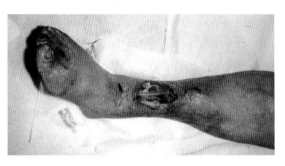

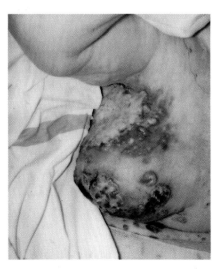

Plate 26 (above) A neuropathic ulcer.
Plate 27 (right) A fungating breast lesion.

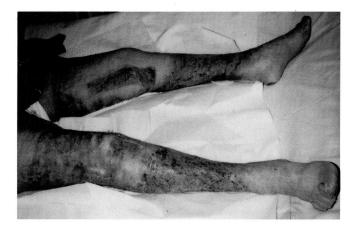

Plate 28 Healed mesh skin grafts.

Plate 29 Drainage of a small haematoma.

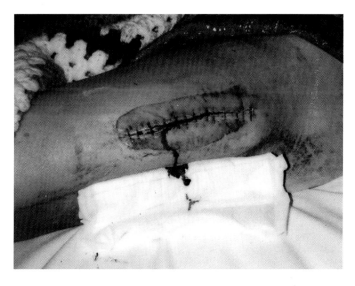

Plate 30 An example of a dehiscent wound.

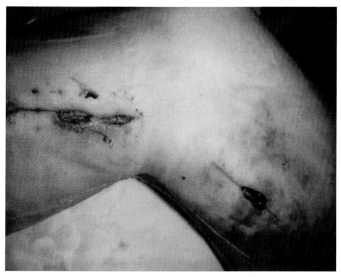

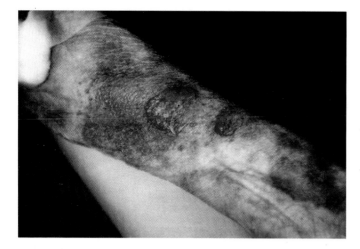

Plate 31 (left) A skin tear or laceration.
Plate 32 (below left) A pretibial laceration.
Plate 33 (bottom left) Taping of a pretibial laceration.

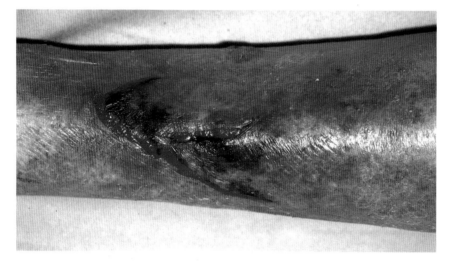

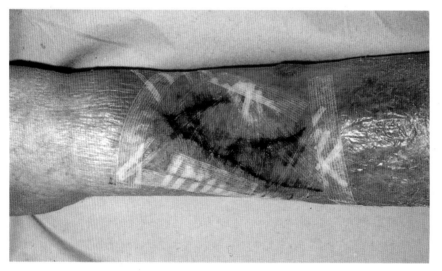

and secrete proteins and growth factors resulting in the generation of a three-dimensional human dermis which can then be used to graft over wound sites. Two brands are currently available: Apligraf® which can be described as cultured human skin equivalent (HSE), and Dermagraft® which consists of tissue-engineered dermis.

Falanga et al. (1998) studied the effect of using a HSE (Apligraf®) on patients with venous ulcers. A total of 275 patients were randomised to HSE and compression, or compression therapy alone. They found a significantly faster healing rate in the HSE group. Gentzkow et al. (1996) carried out a randomised controlled single-blinded trial of 50 patients with diabetic foot ulcers. Patients were allocated to four groups, three different dosages of Dermagraft® or a control group. They found that all three treatment regimens were significantly better than the control. Furthermore after 14 months follow-up there were no recurrences in the Dermagraft® patients. The authors considered this fact to be significant quoting recurrence rates from other studies of from 19.6% to 46% in times less than 12 months.

Grey et al. (1998), reporting on an open study of six patients with neuropathic diabetic foot ulcers, found a positive outcome and considered that there was a definite role for tissue-engineered products in the diabetic foot clinic. Foster et al. (1998) have also reported the early results of a study of diabetic patients with foot ulcers. They found Dermagraft® to be easy to apply and to result in healthy granulating wound beds. Economou et al. (1995) studied the effect of bacterial wound contamination on skin graft viability when using a Dermagraft® and found that it did not affect graft loss.

A variation of HSE is TransCyte® (formally known as Dermagraft-TC®) which is a temporary skin replacement for surgically excised burn wounds requiring grafting. This product is a human fibroblast-derived temporary skin substitute which is removed as epithelialisation occurs. Purdue et al. (1997) report on a randomised study of 66 patients where Dermagraft-TC® was compared with human cadaver allograft for the temporary closure of burn wounds. The skin replacements were removed when clinically indicated and the wound beds were evaluated and prepared for grafting. Overall, Dermagraft-TC® produced a more satisfactory result with respect to ease of removal, less epidermal slough, less bleeding and a greater autograft take.

It is probably too soon to be totally certain of all the benefits, or otherwise, of tissue engineering. However, it is an exciting development which potentially looks to have a wider application than tissue cultures.

4.8 ALTERNATIVE THERAPIES AND WOUND MANAGEMENT

Alternative or complementary therapies have been defined as those therapies that usually lie outside the official health sector (WHO, 1983). Trevelyn and Booth (1994) divided them into three categories in relation to their potential links to nursing (see Table 4.2). Although there is much written in the literature regarding these therapies, there is a paucity of research evidence to demonstrate their place in patient care. Gates (1994) and Vickers (1997) have discussed this problem and suggested the need for a critical appraisal of the literature on the subject.

Table 4.2 Categories of alternative therapies related to nursing.

Category 1: can be incorporated into nursing care

massage
reflexology
aromatherapy
therapeutic touch

Category 2: can be used to some extent by nurses

homeopathy
herbal medicine

Category 3: not usually practised as part of nursing care

acupuncture
osteopathy
chiropractice

One such review has been undertaken by Finch (1997), who appraised the therapy of therapeutic touch, healing by laying on of hands, in relation to wound healing. Its use in nursing was introduced in the USA in the 1970s. It is based on the principle that human beings are energy fields and illness is the result of an imbalance in the energy field. Therapeutic touch focuses on redirecting the energy to restore balance. Finch reviewed five studies of therapeutic touch and wound healing carried out on healthy volunteers by the same researcher. She concluded that therapeutic touch was unreliable and generally ineffective when used to treat wounds. However, it has been shown to be beneficial in treating anxiety (see Chapter 2).

Aromatherapy involves the use of essential oils which are applied to the skin. A variety of oils can be used, depending on the effect required. Unfortunately, there are a number of inconsistencies found in the literature with a variety of contradictory properties being given to the same oil (Vickers, 1997). A recent study by Kite *et al.* (1998) suggests that aromatherapy is effective in reducing anxiety and stress. They assessed 58 cancer patients using a HAD score before and after six sessions of aromatherapy. They found a significant reduction in anxiety and depression at the end of the course of treatment.

There is no doubt that some patients have found alternative therapies helpful. Whether these types of therapies have a role in wound healing remains questionable. There is a real need for the development of high-quality research methodologies to explore the multifaceted nature of these treatments.

REFERENCES

Alvarez, O.M., Dellanoy, O.A. (1987) Moist wound healing. *Paper presented at American Academy of Dermatology.*

Argenta, L.C., Morykwas, M.J. (1997) Vacuum-assisted closure: a new method for wound control and treatment: clinical experience. *Annals of Plastic Surgery,* **38** (6), 563–576.

Arnold, F. (1996) Growth factor treatment for wounds: magic bullets or high-tech hype? in (eds) Cherry, G.W., Gottrup, F., Lawrence, J.C., Moffatt, C.J., Turner, T.D., *Proceedings of the 5th European Conference on Advances in Wound Management.* Macmillan Magazines Ltd, London.

Baxandall, T. (1996) Healing cavity wounds with negative pressure. *Nursing Standard,* **11** (6), 49–51.

Becker, G.D. (1986) Identification and management of the patient at high risk of wound infection. *Head and Neck Surgery,* **8**, 205–210.

Blackburn, J.H., Boemi, L., Hall, W.W., Jeffords, K., Hauck, R.M., Banducci, D.R., Graham, W.P. III (1998) Negative-pressure dressings as a bolster for skin grafts. *Annals of Plastic Surgery,* **40** (5), 453–457.

Bloomfield, S.F., Sizer, T.J. (1985) Eusol BPC and other hypochlorite formulations used in hospitals. *Pharmaceutical Journal,* **253**, 153–157.

Bond, C.J. (1915) The application of strong antiseptics to wounds. *British Medical Journal,* **March 6**, 405–406.

Brannen, A.L., Still, J., Haynes, M., Orlet, H., Rosenblum, F., Law, E., Thompson, W.O. (1997) A randomised prospective trial of hyperbaric oxygen in a referral burn centre population. *American Surgery,* **63** (3), 205–208.

Brennan, S.S., Foster, M.E., Leaper, D.J. (1986) Antiseptic toxicity in wounds healing by second intention. *Journal of Hospital Infection,* **8** (3), 263–267.

Brennan, S.S., Leaper, D.J. (1985) The effect of antiseptics on the healing wound: a study using the rabbit ear chamber. *British Journal of Surgery,* **72** (10), 780–782.

British Medical Association Board of Science and Education (1993) *Clinical Hyperbaric Medicine Facilities in the UK.* British Medical Association, London.

Bux, M., Baig, M.K., Rodrigues, E., Armstrong, D., Brown, A. (1997) Antibody response to topical streptokinase. *Journal of Wound Care,* **6** (2), 70–73.

Church, J.C.T. (1996) Blow-fly larvae as agents of debridement in chronically infected wounds, in (eds) Cherry, G.W., Gottrup, F., Lawrence, J.C., Moffatt, C.J., Turner, T.D., *Proceedings of the 5th European Conference on Advances in Wound Management.* Macmillan Magazines Ltd, London.

Ciaravino, M.E., Friedell, M.L., Kammerlocher, T.C. (1996) Is hyperbaric oxygen a useful adjunct in the management of problem lower extremity wounds? *Annals of Vascular Surgery,* **10** (6), 558–562.

Coady, M.S. (1992) Eusol: the continuing controversy. *British Medical Journal,* **304** (6842), 1636.

Cookson, B. (1998) The emergence of mupirocin resistance: a challenge to infection control and antibiotic prescribing practice. *Journal of Antimicrobial Chemotherapy,* **41** (1), 11–18.

Daltrey, D.C., Cunliffe, W.J. (1981) A double-blind study of the effects of Benzol peroxide 20% and Eusol and liquid paraffin on the microbial flora of leg ulcers. *Acta Dermatology and Venereology,* **61**, 575–577.

D'Arcy, P.F. (1972) Drugs on the skin: a clinical and pharmaceutical problem. *Pharmaceutical Journal,* **209**, 491–492.

Deng, S., Sang, J., Cao, L. (1995) The effects of mupirocin on burn wounds with *Staphylococcus aureus* infection. *Chung Hua Cheng Hsing Shao Shang Wai Ko Tsa Chih,* **11** (1), 45–48.

Dubranski, S., Duncan, S.E., Harkiss, A., Ball, A., Robertson, D. (1983) Topical applications in pressure sore therapy. *British Journal of Pharmaceutical Practice,* **5** (5), 10.

Duin, N., Sutcliffe, J. (1992) *A History of Medicine.* Simon & Schuster, London.

Eaglstein, W.H. (1985) Experiences with biosynthetic dressings. *Journal of the American Academy of Dermatology*, **12**, 434–440.

Economou, T.P., Rosenquist, M.D., Lewis R.W. II, Kealey, G.P. (1995) An experimental study to determine the effects of Dermagraft on skin graft viability in the presence of bacterial wound contamination. *Journal of Burn Care Rehabilitation*, **16** (1), 267–70.

Falanga, V., Marolis, D., Alvarez, O., Auletta, M., Maggiocomo, F., Altman, M. *et al.* (1998) Rapid healing of venous ulcers and lack of clinical rejection with an allogeneic cultured human skin equivalent. *Archives of Dermatology*, **134**, 293–300.

Finch, A. (1997) Therapeutic touch and wound healing. *Journal of Wound Care*, **6** (10), 501–504.

Forrest, R.D. (1982) Early history of wound treatment. *Journal of the Royal Society of Medicine*, **75**, 198–205.

Foster, A.V.M., McColgan, M., Edmonds, M.E. (1998) Dermagraft: a new treatment for diabetic foot wounds, in (eds) Leaper, D., Dealey, C., Franks, P.J., Hofman, D., Moffat, C.J., *Proceedings of the 7th European Conference on Advances in Wound Management*. Macmillan Magazines Ltd, London.

Freidman, S., Su, D.W.P. (1983) Hydrocolloid occlusive dressing management of leg ulcers. *Archives of Dermatology*, **120**, 1329–1331.

Gates, B. (1994) The use of complementary and alternative therapies in health care: a selective review of the literature and discussion of the implications for nurse practitioners and health-care managers. *Journal of Clinical Nursing*, **3** (1), 43–47.

Gentzkow, G.D., Iswaki, S.D., Hershon, K.S. *et al.* (1996) Use of Dermagraft, a cultured human dermis, to treat diabetic foot ulcers. *Diabetes Care*, **19** (4), 350–354.

Gilchrist, B. (1997) Should iodine be reconsidered in wound management? *Journal of Wound Care*, **6** (3), 148–150.

Graber, R.P., Vistnes, L., Pardoes, R. (1975) The effect of commonly used antiseptics on wound healing. *Plastic and Reconstructive Surgery*, **55**, 472–6.

Grey, J.E., Lowe, G., Bale, S., Harding, K.G. (1998) The use of Dermagraft in the treatment of long-standing and difficult-to-heal diabetic foot ulcers, in (eds) Leaper, D.J., Cherry, G., Cockbill, S., Dealey, C., Flanagan, M., Hofman, D. *et al.*, *Proceedings of the EWMA/Journal of Wound Care Spring Meeting: New Approaches to the Management of Chronic Wounds*. Macmillan Magazines Ltd., London.

Hall-Angeras, M., Brandberg, A., Falk, A., Seeman, T. (1992) Comparison between sterile saline and tap water for the cleansing of acute traumatic soft tissue wounds. *European Journal of Surgery*, **158**, 347–350.

Herzog, W. (1915) German experiences. The dangers of tincture of iodine as a first-aid dressing. *British Medical Journal*, **March 6**, 441–442.

Humzah, M.D., Marshall, J., Breach, N.M. (1996) Eusol: the plastic surgeon's choice? *Journal of the Royal College of Surgeons in Edinburgh*, **41**, 269–270.

Johnson, A. (1987) Wound care, packing cavity wounds. *Nursing Times*, **83** (36), 59–62.

Jones, M., Thomas, S. (1997) Wound cleansing – a therapy revisited. *Journal of Tissue Viability*, **7** (4), 119–121.

Kakibuchi, M., Hosokawa, K., Fujikawa, M., Yoshikawa, K. (1996) The use of cultured epidermal cell sheets in skin grafting. *Journal of Wound Care*, 5 (10), 487–490.

Kaufman, C., Hirshowitz, B. (1983) Treatment of chronic leg ulcers with Opsite. *Chirurgica Plastica*, **7**, 211–215.

Kearney, J.N., Arain, T., Holland, K.T. (1988) Antimicrobial properties of antiseptic impregnated dressings. *Journal of Hospital Infection*, **11** (1), 68–76.

Kirkpatrick, J.J.R., Naylor, I.L. (1997) Ulcer management in medieval England. *Journal of Wound Care*, **6** (7), 350–352.

Kite, S.M., Maher, E.J., Anderson, K., Young, T., Young, J., Howells, N., Bradburn, J. (1998) Development of an aromatherapy service at a cancer centre. *Palliative Medicine*, **12** (3), 171–180.

Knighton, D.R., Ciresi, K., Fiegal, V.D., Schumerth, S., Butler, E., Cerrs, F. (1990) Stimulation of repair in chronic non-healing cutaneous ulcers using platelet-derived wound healing formula. *Surgery, Gynaecology & Obstetrics*, **170**, 56–60.

Kumagai, N., Oshima, H., Tanabe, M., Ishida, H., Uchikoshi, T. (1997) Favourable donor site for epidermal cultivation for the treatment of burn scars with autologous cultured epithelium. *Annals of Plastic Surgery*, **38** (5), 506–513.

Lawrence, J.C. (1987) A century after Gamgee. *Burns*, **13** (1), 77–79.

Leaper, D.J. (1992) Eusol. *British Medical Journal*, **304** (6832), 930–931.

Lineaweaver, W., Howard, R., Soucy, D., McMorris, S., Freeman, J., Crain, C. *et al.* (1985) Topical antimicrobial toxicity. *Archives of Surgery*, **120**, 267–270.

McLure, A.R., Gordon J. (1992) In-vitro evaluation of povidone-iodine and chlorhexidine against methicillin resistant *Staphylococcus aureus*. *Journal of Hospital Infection*, **21**, 291–299.

May, S.R. (1984) Physiology, immunology and clinical efficacy of an adherent polyurethane wound dressing Opsite, in (ed) Wise, D.L., *Burn Wound Coverings*, Vol. II. CRC Press, Boca Raton.

Mayo-Robson, A.W. (1915) Hints on war surgery. *British Journal of Dermatology*, July 24, 136.

Meade, R.H. (1968) *An Introduction to the History of General Surgery*. W.B. Saunders & Co., Philadelphia.

Merchant, J. (1988) Aseptic technique reconsidered. *Care, Science and Practice*, **6** (3), 74–77.

Millward, J. (1989) Assessment of wound management in a Care of the Elderly Unit. *Care, Science and Practice*, **7** (2), 47–49.

Morgan, D. (1993) Is there still a role for antiseptics? *Journal of Tissue Viability*, **3** (3), 80–84.

Morgan, D. (1995) Myiasis: the rise and fall of maggot therapy. *Journal of Tissue Viability*, **5** (2), 43–51.

Murray, Y. (1988) An investigation into the care of wounds in a health authority. *Care Science and Practice*, **6** (4), 97–102.

Myers, J.A. (1982) Modern plastic surgical dressings. *Health and Social Services Journal*, **92**, 336–337.

Myers, S.R., Grady, J., Soranzo, C., Sanders, R., Green, C., Leigh, I.M., Navsaria, H.A. (1997) A hyaluronic acid membrane delivery system for cultured keratinocytes: clinical 'take' rates in the porcine kerato-dermal model. *Journal of Burn Care Rehabilitation*, **18**, 214–222.

Neovius, E.B., Lind, M.G., Lind, F.G. (1997) Hyperbaric oxygen therapy for wound complications after surgery in the irradiated head and neck: a review of the literature and a report of 15 consecutive patients. *Head and Neck*, **19** (4), 315–322.

O'Toole, E.A., Goel, M., Woodley, D.T. (1996) Hydrogen peroxide inhibits human keratinocyte migration. *Dermatology Surgery*, **22** (6), 525–529.

Pizzorno, R., Bonini, F., Donelli, A., Stubinski, R., Medica, M., Carmignani, G. (1997) Hyperbaric oxygen therapy in the treatment of Fournier's disease in 11 male patients. *Journal of Urology*, **158** (3 Pt 1), 837–840.

Popp, A.J. (1995) Crossroads at Salerno: Eldridge Campbell and the writings of Teodorico Borgognoni on wound healing. *Journal of Neurosurgery*, **83**, 174–179.

Purdue, G.F., Hunt, J.L., Still, J.M. Jr, Law, E.J., Herndon, D.N., Goldfarb, I.W., *et al.* (1997) A multicentre clinical trial of a biosynthetic skin replacement, Dermagraft-TC, compared with cryopreserved human cadaver skin for temporary coverage of excised burn wounds. *Journal of Burn Care Rehabilitation,* **18** (1 Pt 1), 52–57.

Reynolds, J.E.F. (ed) (1982) *Martindale: The Extra Pharmacopoeia,* 28th edn. The Pharmaceutical Press, London.

Rode, H., Hanslo, D., de Wet, P.M., Millar, A.J., Cywes, S. (1989) Efficacy of mupirocin in methicillin-resistant *Staphylococcus aureus* burn wound infection. *Antimicrobial Agents and Chemotherapy,* **33** (8), 1358–1361.

Russ, M., Fleischmann, W., Lang, E. (1997) Vacuum sealing technique for the treatment of acute and chronic infections, in (eds) Leaper, D.J., Cherry, G.W., Dealey, C., Lawrence, J.C., Turner, T.D., *Proceedings of the 6th European Conference on Advances in Wound Management.* Macmillan Magazines Ltd, London.

Russell, A.D., Hugo, W.B., Ayliffe, G.A.J. (1982) *Principles and Practice of Disinfection, Preservation and Sterilisation.* Blackwell Scientific Publications, London.

Sinclair, R.D., Ryan, T.J. (1993) A great war for antiseptics. *Wound Management,* **4** (1), 16–18.

Sleigh, J.W., Linter, S.P.K. (1985) Hazards of hydrogen peroxide. *British Medical Journal,* **291**, 1706.

Spencer, M.J., Herrick, S.E., Shah, M., Greenwood, J., McCollum, C.M., Boulton, A.J.M. *et al.* (1996) Growth factor therapy: redressing the balance, in (eds) Cherry, G.W., Gottrup, F., Lawrence, J.C., Moffatt, C.J., Turner, T.D., *Proceedings of the 5th European Conference on Advances in Wound Management.* Macmillan Magazines Ltd, London.

Tatnall, F.M., Leigh, I.M., Gibson, J.R. (1990) Comparative study of antiseptic toxicity on basal keratinocytes, transformed human keratinocytes and fibroblasts. *Skin Pharmacology,* **3** (3), 157–163.

Teot, L., Fabre, J.M., Cherenfant, E., Hussenet, P. (1997) Abdominal parietal defect treated using vacuum assisted closure, in (eds) Leaper, D.J., Cherry, G.W., Dealey, C., Lawrence, J.C., Turner, T.D., *Proceedings of the 6th European Conference on Advances in Wound Management.* Macmillan Magazines Ltd, London.

Thomas, S. (1986) Milton and the treatment of burns. *Pharmaceutical Journal,* **236**, 128–129.

Thomas, S. (1990) Eusol revisited. *Dressing Times,* **3** (1), 3–4.

Thomas, S., Jones, M., Shutler, S., Jones, S. (1996) Using larvae in modern wound management. *Journal of Wound Care,* **5** (2), 60–69.

Thomlinson, D. (1987) To clean or not to clean. *Nursing Times,* **83** (9), 71–75.

Trevelyn, J. (1997) Spirit of the beehive. *Nursing Times,* **93** (7), 72–74.

Trevelyn, J., Booth, B. (1994) *Complementary Medicine for Nurses, Midwives & Health Visitors.* Macmillan Press, London.

Trilla, A., Miro, J.M. (1995) Identifying high risk patients for *Staphylococcus aureus* infections: skin and soft tissue infections. *Journal of Chemotherapy,* **7** (Suppl. 3), 37–43.

Turner, T.D. (1986) Recent advances in wound management products, in (eds) Turner, T.D., Schmidt, R.J., Harding, K.G., *Advances in Wound Management.* John Wiley and Sons, Chichester.

Vickers, A. (1997) Yes, but how do we know it's true? Knowledge claims in massage and aromatherapy. *Complementary Therapy in Nursing & Midwifery,* **3** (3), 63–65.

Voinchet, V., Berret, M., Favoli, P., Casanova, D., Legre, R., Magalon, G. (1997) Vacuum-assisted closure: wound healing by negative pressure, in (eds) Leaper, D.J., Cherry,

G.W., Dealey, C., Lawrence, J.C., Turner, T.D., *Proceedings of the 6th European Conference on Advances in Wound Management.* Macmillan Magazines Ltd, London.

Walsh, M. and Ford, P. (1989) *Nursing Rituals, Research and Rational Actions.* Heinemann Nursing, Oxford.

WHO (1983) *Traditional Medicine and Health-Care Coverage.* World Health Organisation, Geneva.

Winter, G.D. (1962) Formation of the scab and the rate of epithelialisation of superficial wounds in the skin of the domestic pig. *Nature,* **193**, 293.

Wright, K.A., Nadire, K.B., Busto, P., Tubo, R., McPherson, J.M., Wentworth, B.M. (1998) Alternative delivery of keratinocytes using polyurethane membrane and the implications for its use in the treatment of full-thickness burn injury. *Burns,* **24** (1), 7–17.

Zamboni, W.A., Wong, H.P., Stephenson, L.L., Pfeifer, M.A. (1997) Evaluation of hyperbaric oxygen for diabetic wounds: a prospective study. *Undersea Hyperbaric Medicine,* **24** (3), 175–179.

Zimmerman, L.M., Veith, I. (1961) *Great Ideas in the History of Surgery.* Wilkins & Wilkins Co., Baltimore.

Chapter 5
The Management of Patients with Chronic Wounds

5.1 INTRODUCTION

A chronic wound was defined by Fowler (1990) as one where there is tissue deficit as the result of longstanding injury or insult or frequent recurrence. Despite medical or nursing care chronic wounds do not heal easily. They are more likely to occur in the elderly or those with multisystem problems. This section will consider the care of patients with pressure sores, leg ulcers and fungating wounds.

Chronic wounds cause much discomfort and pain. A multidisciplinary approach is needed for their management and prevention. Nurses can play an important role in the team as they usually have the most contact with the patient. An essential part of this role is communication and co-operation across the disciplines. Healing is not possible for all chronic wounds and in these cases the goal is to assist the patient to achieve the maximum independence and function possible.

5.2 THE PREVENTION AND MANAGEMENT OF PRESSURE SORES

Pressure sores are also called 'pressure ulcers', 'bed sores' and 'decubitus ulcers'. A pressure sore can be described as localised damage to the skin caused by disruption of the blood supply to the area, usually caused by pressure, shear or friction, or a combination of any of these. There has not been a national survey of pressure sore prevalence in the UK; however, a survey by O'Dea (1995) of over 8000 patients found that 18.6% of hospital patients had pressure sores. A national survey in the USA found a pressure sore prevalence of 10.1% in acute hospital patients (Barczak *et al.*, 1997). Barrois *et al.* (1998) reviewed the epidemiology of pressure sores in countries across Europe and found that the prevalence was between 6% and 9% in France, Spain, Greece and Sweden.

For many years pressure sores were seen as a failure of care, in particular, the result of bad nursing. Florence Nightingale (1861) considered that good nursing could prevent them, whereas a very influential French doctor called Jean-Martin Charcot (1825–1893) believed that doctors could do nothing about pressure sores. As a result, pressure sores became a very emotive issue and were referred to by doctors as 'a nursing problem' and by nurses with comments such as 'we do not have pressure sores here'.

This attitude is changing. A document published by the Department of Health stated that pressure sores should be considered a key indicator of the quality of care provided by a hospital (DoH, 1993). There is a much greater awareness that all healthcare professionals need to be involved in pressure sore prevention (Culley, 1998). A number of multidisciplinary societies have been formed such as the Tissue Viability Society and the European Pressure Ulcer Advisory Panel with the intent of expanding knowledge and supporting good practice.

5.2.1 The aetiology of pressure sores

Pressure sores are caused by a combination of factors both outside and inside the patient.

External factors

There are three external factors which can cause pressure sores either on their own or in any combination of the three. They are pressure, shear and friction.

Pressure is the most important factor in pressure sore development. When the soft tissue of the body is compressed between a bony prominence and a hard surface causing pressures greater than capillary pressure, localised ischaemia occurs. The normal body response to such pressure is to shift position so the pressure is redistributed. When pressure is relieved a red area appears over the bony prominence. This is called reactive hyperaemia and is the result of a temporarily increased blood supply to the area, removing waste products and bringing oxygen and nutrients. It is a normal physiological response.

Capillary pressure is generally described as being approximately 32 mmHg, based on the research of Landis (1931). His research was carried out on young, healthy students. He found the average arteriolar pressure was 32 mmHg, but the average pressure in the venules was 12 mmHg. There is also a certain amount of tissue tension which resists deformation. It is not uncommon for interface pressures of around 30–40 mmHg to be seen as 'safe'. This is not always correct. Ageing causes a reduction in the numbers of elastic fibres in the tissues, resulting in reduced tissue tension. In situations where the blood pressure is artificially lowered, such as during some types of surgery, capillary pressure is also likely to be lower. In these circumstances, very little pressure is required to cause capillary occlusion. Ek *et al.* (1987) found that a pressure of only 11 mmHg was necessary to cause capillary occlusion in some hemiplegic patients.

If unrelieved pressure persists for a long period of time, tissue necrosis will follow. Prolonged pressure causes distortion of the soft tissues and results in destruction of tissue close to the bone. A cone-shaped sore is created, with the widest part of the cone close to the bone and the narrowest on the body surface. Thus, the visible sore fails to reveal the true extent of tissue damage.

The bony prominences which are most vulnerable to pressure sore development are sometimes referred to as the pressure areas. They include: the sacrum, ischial tuberosities, trochanters, heels and elbows (see Fig. 5.1).

Shear forces can deform and disrupt tissue and so damage the blood vessels.

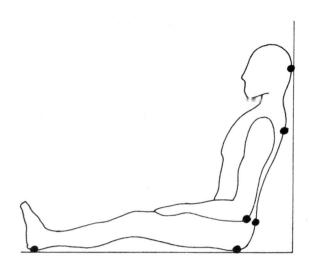

Fig. 5.1 The bony prominences or pressure areas.

Gebhardt (1995) argues that pressure is rarely applied uniformly and that the subsequent distortion leads to shearing. Shearing may occur if the patient slides down the bed. The skeleton and tissues nearest to it move, but the skin on the buttocks remains still. One of the main culprits of shearing is the back-rest of the bed which encourages sliding. Chairs which fail to maintain a good posture may also cause shearing.

Friction occurs when two surfaces rub together. The commonest cause is when the patient is dragged rather than lifted across the bed. It causes the top layers of epithelial cells to be scraped off. 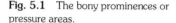 Moisture exacerbates the effect of friction. Moisture may be found on a patient's skin as a result of excessive sweating or urinary incontinence.

Internal factors

The human body is frequently subjected to some or all of the external factors, but does not automatically develop pressure sores. The determining factor(s) come from within the patient.

General health is important as the body can withstand greater external pressure in health than when sick. Bliss (1990) suggests that the acutely ill are particularly vulnerable. Although the reasons for this are not certain, Bliss suggests some precipitating factors including pain, low blood pressure, heart failure, the use of sedatives, vasomotor failure, peripheral vasoconstriction due to shock and others.

Age has been shown to be a major factor in the development of pressure sores. David *et al.* (1983) carried out a pressure sore prevalence survey of 20 health districts from within four health regions. They found that 85% of the patients with pressure sores were over 65 years old. A survey by Nyquist and Hawthorn (1987) found that within one health authority 47% of patients with pressure sores were on wards for the elderly.

As people age, their skin becomes thinner and less elastic. In part, this is because the collagen in the dermis reduces in quantity and quality. Collagen provides a buffer which helps to prevent disruption of the microcirculation (Krouskop, 1983). There may be wasting of the overall body mass, resulting in loose folds of skin. There is also an increased likelihood of chronic illnesses or diseases developing, many of which may also predispose to pressure sore development. Once a sore occurs it is much harder to heal in an older person than a young one (see Chapter 2).

Reduced mobility can affect the ability to relieve pressure effectively, if at all. It also predisposes to shearing and friction if the patient is confined to a bed or chair. General prevalence surveys such as those of David *et al.* (1983) and Nyquist and Hawthorn (1987) found reduced mobility to be a factor for many patients with pressure sores. Versluysen (1986) studied 100 patients over 60 years old with a fractured femur and found a prevalence of 66%. This study was replicated by Nyquist and Hawthorn (1988) who found a prevalence of 42.3%.

Exton-Smith and Sherwin (1961) studied the number of movements made by 50 elderly patients during the night. A strong relationship was found between those with reduced movement and the development of pressure sores. Reduced movement during sleep may be associated with a variety of drugs such as hypnotics, anxiolytics, antidepressants, opioid analgesics and antihistamines. Berlowitz and Wilking (1989) studied a variety of factors in patients with pressure sores, and patients developing pressure sores, and found that reduced mobility was significantly associated with pressure sores in both groups. Brandeis *et al.* (1994) also found reduced mobility to be a significant factor in a study involving nursing home patients.

Another aspect of reduced mobility is that of the patient undergoing major surgery. Operations may last many hours while the patient lies immobile on the hard operating table. Mobility may also be reduced in the immediate postoperative period because of the effects of the anaesthetic, pain, analgesia, infusions or drains. Today, very sophisticated surgery is carried out, often on older patients as well. The risks of pressure sore development associated with such surgery are consequently increased.

Reduced mobility may also be associated with neurological deficit, such as a patient with paraplegia, but this is not always so. A diabetic patient may suffer from neuropathy without loss of mobility. Neurological deficit may be associated with strokes, multiple sclerosis, diabetes, and spinal cord injury or degeneration. Loss of sensation means the patient is unaware of the need to relieve pressure, even if able to do so. Dealey (1991a) found that neurological deficit was a common factor in those patients with pressure sores found in a survey of a teaching hospital. Kabagambe *et al.* (1994) took 10 patients with spinal cord injury and compared them with 11 healthy subjects. They found an impaired reactive hyperaemia response in those with spinal cord injury.

Reduced nutritional status impairs the elasticity of the skin. Long term it will lead to anaemia and a reduction of oxygen to the tissues. Pinchkofsky-Devin and Kaminski (1986) assessed the nutritional status of 232 patients in a nursing home; of these, 117 patients had mild-to-moderate malnutrition and 17 had severe malnutrition. Although none of the other patients had pressure sores, they were present in all the 17 severely malnourished patients. Cullum and Clark (1992) carried out a study of intrinsic factors associated with pressure sores in elderly people. They found that serum protein concentrations were significantly lower in those patients admitted with pressure sores and those who developed sores when compared with patients who did not have pressure sores. Berlowitz and Wilking (1989) and Brandeis *et al.* (1994) also found impaired nutritional intake a factor in pressure sore development. The factors which may lead to malnutrition are discussed in Chapter 2.

Body weight should also be considered. Very emaciated patients have no 'padding' over bony prominences. They have less protection against pressure. On the other hand, very obese patients are difficult to move. Unless great care is taken, they may be dragged rather than lifted in the bed. Another problem of the obese patient is that moisture from sweating may become trapped between the rolls of fat causing maceration. Both of these types of patient may also have a poor nutritional status.

Incontinence of urine can contribute to maceration of the skin and thus increase the risk of friction. Constant washing removes natural body oils, drying the skin. In a pressure sore prevalence survey of Greater Glasgow, Jordan and Clark (1977) found 15.5% of patients with pressure sores to be incontinent of urine and 39.7% to have faecal incontinence. Schnelle *et al.* (1997) found incontinence to be related to blanching erythema, an early indicator of pressure damage. Factors that may be associated with urinary incontinence include the use of diuretics or sedatives. Diarrhoea may cause incontinence in the elderly or immobile patient. It is a side-effect found with the use of some antibiotics.

Poor blood supply to the periphery lowers the local capillary pressure and causes malnutrition in the tissues. It may be caused by disease, such as heart disease, peripheral vascular disease or diabetes. Drugs, such as beta-blockers and inotropic sympathomimetics, may cause peripheral vasoconstriction. These drugs may be used following cardiac surgery when the patient is already suffering from reduced mobility. Blood flow may also be affected during surgery. Sanada *et al.* (1997) measured blood flow during surgery in the skin over the iliac crest and sacrum. They found a 500% increase in flow in those patients who did not develop pressure sores, but a drop in flow in those who later developed pressure sores.

Dealey (1997) cited a number of external factors which can exacerbate the internal factors discussed above. They include:

- inappropriate positioning, which may increase pressure or shear;
- restrictions to movement such as lying for long periods on a trolley;
- lying for long periods in one position on hard surfaces such as the X-ray table;
- poor lifting and handling techniques increase the risk of friction and shear;
- poor hygiene which leaves the skin surface moist from urine, faeces or sweat;
- drugs such as sedatives which make the patient drowsy and less likely to move.

5.2.2 The cost of pressure sores

The true cost of pressure sores is impossible to calculate. There is the untold cost in terms of pain and suffering to the patient as well as the cost to the health service.

There are few official data in the UK. The Department of Health commissioned a report into the costs of pressure sores by Touche Ross & Co. (1993). Their work produced estimates rather than precise figures using a mythical 600-bed hospital. They worked on high and low costs for both prevention and treatment (see Table 5.1). It can be argued that their costings were flawed as they included the cost of a clinical nurse specialist in tissue viability in the cost of prevention but not for treatment costs. They also suggested that staff spent more time on preventing a patient from developing a pressure sore than treating a patient with a sore. Most nurses would take issue with this conclusion.

Table 5.1 The costs of pressure sores.

	Prevention	Treatment
Low cost	£644 797	£644 661
High cost	£2 709 878	£1 153 498

From Touche Ross & Co. (1993).

Several others have looked at some aspect of costings, one of the most often quoted is a study by Hibbs. Hibbs (1988) calculated that the cost of treating one patient with a deep sacral pressure sore was £25 905.58. This patient was in hospital for 180 days. A further calculation looked at the 'opportunity costs'. Opportunity costs describe what has been foregone because of specific circumstances. For example, because of the extended stay in hospital of this patient, the opportunity to carry out 16 routine hip or knee replacements was lost. Similar calculations can also be made looking at standard days and standard costs. A critique of this work was published by two economists nine years later (Brooks & Thompson, 1997). They support Hibbs's approach and regret that there have been few economic appraisals in relation to pressure sore prevention. Dealey (1993) noted the cost of treating one patient to be just over £22 000. The cost of a suitable mattress to prevent further breakdown after discharge was £450 – indicating that prevention is cheaper than cure. Clough (1994) drew a similar conclusion in his study. He found that it cost £320 per patient to treat patients in an intensive care unit with pressure sores whereas it cost £150 per patient for prevention.

Some studies have looked at length of stay as a way of assessing pressure sore costs. Lapsley and Vogels (1996) looked at the cost of pressure sores in patients who had undergone surgery either for hip replacement or coronary artery bypass graft. They found a significantly longer stay for those patients who developed pressure sores compared with those who did not. Stordeur et al. (1998) also studied patients undergoing cardiovascular surgery. They found that the total length of stay was longer by a mean of six days for those who developed pressure sores.

Another cost that has to be taken into consideration is that of litigation. Tingle (1997) describes a number of legal cases where the patient or their families were awarded damages ranging from £3500 to £12 500. In all of these cases there is a chronicle of incompetence and negligent care. In some instances the pressure sore directly contributed to the patient's death. Allied to this there is often inadequate assessment and poor documentation.

5.2.3 The prevention of pressure sores

Although it is a truism, as far as pressure sores are concerned, prevention is better than cure. Waterlow (1988) suggests that 95% of all pressure sores could be prevented. The document *Health of the Nation* (DoH, 1992) calls for an annual reduction of 5–10%. in the incidence of pressure sores. To this end most trusts now have pressure sore prevention policies. There is also a move towards the development of evidence-based guidelines to provide a framework from which local policies may be developed. European pressure sore prevention guidelines have recently been published and will provide a useful framework for discussing prevention (European Pressure Ulcer Advisory Panel, 1998). The guidelines can be divided into sections on risk assessment, improving tissue tolerance, pressure relief and education. Each section is cited in full in Tables 5.2–5.5.

Table 5.2 European Pressure Ulcer Advisory Panel guidelines on pressure ulcer prevention.

---

(1) Identify 'at risk' individuals needing prevention and the specific factors placing them at risk

---

- We believe that there are a number of issues associated with risk assessment tools. Risk assessment should be as an adjunct to clinical judgement and not as a tool in isolation from other clinical features (C).
- There should be clarification of a full risk assessment of patients to include: general medical condition, skin assessment, mobility, moistness and incontinence, nutrition and pain (C).
- All strategies related to pressure damage should always be based on the best available evidence.
- Assessment of risk should be more than just the use of an appropriate risk assessment tool and should not lead to a prescriptive and inflexible approach to patient care (C). While risk assessment should be performed immediately on entry into a care episode, this assessment may take time to fully complete if information is not readily available (C). Assessment should be ongoing and frequency of reassessment should be dependent on change in the patient's condition.

The letters A–C in Tables 5.2–5.5 refer to the grading recommendations of the European Pressure Ulcer Advisory Panel (1998). For definitions of each grade, see Table 8.3.

(1) Identify 'at risk' individuals needing prevention and the specific factors placing them at risk.
Too often, risk assessment is just seen as using a risk calculator to determine the patient's score and then following a 'recipe' of care. Risk calculators should be part of the assessment process. However, assessment should also include: general medical condition, a nutritional assessment, skin assessment, identification of any incontinence and the effect that this may have on the skin and also the level of mobility.

There are a number of risk calculators available. The earliest that was developed was the Norton Score (Norton *et al.*, 1975). Subsequently other scores have been

Table 5.3 European Pressure Ulcer Advisory Panel guidelines on pressure ulcer prevention.

(2) Maintain and improve tissue tolerance to pressure in order to prevent injury

- Skin condition should be documented daily and any changes should be recorded as soon as they are observed. Inspection must be documented. Initial skin assessment should take into account the following:
  I. Bony prominences (sacrum, heels, hips, ankles, elbows, occiput) to identify early signs of pressure damage.
  II. Identify the condition of the skin: dryness, cracking, erythema, maceration, fragility, heat and induration (C).
  Every effort should be made to optimise the condition of the patient's skin. Assessment of patients with dark or tanned skin is especially difficult (C).
- Avoid excessive rubbing over bony prominences as this does not prevent pressure damage and may cause additional damage (C).
- Find the sources of excess moisture due to incontinence, perspiration or wound drainage and eliminate this, where possible. When moisture cannot be controlled interventions that can assist in preventing skin damage should be used (C).
- Skin injury due to friction and shear forces should be minimised through correct positioning, transferring and repositioning techniques.
- Following assessment, nutritionally compromised individuals should have a plan of appropriate support and/or supplementation that meets individual needs and is consistent with overall goals of therapy (C).
- As the patient's condition improves the potential for improving mobility and activity status exists, rehabilitation efforts may be instituted if consistent with overall goals of therapy. Maintaining activity level, mobility and range of movement is an appropriate goal for most individuals (C).
- All interventions and outcomes should be documented (C).

developed. Probably the most widely used within UK hospitals is the Waterlow Score (see Fig. 5.2 (Waterlow, 1985)). This calculator considers a wider range of variables than Norton. The scoring is also reversed so that the higher the score, the higher the risk. It has the advantage of dividing the degree of risk into categories; 'at risk', 'high risk' and 'very high risk'. These can be useful when considering the use of appropriate support systems. Waterlow included suggestions for preventive measures on the reverse of the card. The Braden Score (Bergstrom *et al.*, 1985) is widely used in the USA. It has been demonstrated to have greater sensitivity and specificity than other scales, but only if used by registered nurses (Bergstrom *et al.*, 1987).

Risk calculators have been judged according to their sensitivity and specificity. Sensitivity relates to the percentage of patients predicted to develop pressure sores who have gone on to develop them. Specificity is defined as the percentage of patients deemed not to be at risk who do not develop pressure sores (Anthony, 1996). Bridel (1993a) found that the Waterlow Score had a high sensitivity but a lower specificity whereas the reverse was true for the Braden Score. However, the effect of nursing care needs to be taken into account, as it may affect the success of the calculator. Deeks (1996) suggests that where sensitivity and specificity appear to be poor it is often in settings where effective prevention methods are being used.

Despite the criticisms that can be made of the risk calculators, there is benefit in

Table 5.4 European Pressure Ulcer Advisory Panel guidelines on pressure ulcer prevention.

---

(3) Protect against the adverse effects of external mechanical forces: pressure, friction and shear

---

- Any individual who is assessed to be at risk of developing pressure ulcers should be repositioned if it is medically safe to do so (B).
- Frequency of repositioning should be consistent with overall goals (C).
- Documentation to record repositioning should be completed. Correct positioning and support is important to minimise friction and shear in both bed and chair (C).
- Correct positioning or devices such as pillows or foam wedges should be used to keep bony prominences (e.g. knees, heels or ankles) from direct contact with one another in accordance with a written plan (C). Care should be taken to ensure that these do not interfere with the action of any other pressure relieving support systems in use (C).
- When repositioning patients, do so in such a way as to minimise the impact on bony prominences (C).
- Devices to assist manual handling should be used during transfer and positioning of patients to minimise shear forces for those patients who require assistance in movement, in accordance with EU manual handling regulations.
- In all care settings, individuals considered to be at risk of developing pressure ulcers should have a personalised written prevention plan which may include a pressure redistributing device (A).
- Patients at risk of developing pressure ulcers because of the time spent sitting in a chair should be allocated a chair of the correct height in addition to a pressure relieving device (B).
- Any person who is acutely ill and at risk of developing a pressure ulcer should avoid uninterrupted sitting out of bed (B). The period of time should be defined in the individualised care plan, but generally not more than two hours (B). Individuals, where appropriate, should be encouraged to reposition themselves if this is possible (B).
- Individuals at risk from pressure ulcers who are likely to spend substantial periods of time in a chair or wheelchair should generally be provided with a pressure redistributing device (B). Individuals who are able should be taught to redistribute weight every 15 minutes (C).

---

using a systematic method of identifying and assessing patients at risk of pressure sore development. Flanagan (1997) stresses the importance of assessing patients regularly rather than just at an initial assessment. It should also be noted that once a patient is identified as being at risk appropriate preventive action must follow. Failure to do so would be a failure in the duty of care that each nurse has to her patients.

(2) Maintain and improve tissue tolerance to pressure in order to prevent injury.

There is a natural resilience in skin which enables the healthy individual to overcome many of the problems of friction or shear met in everyday life. It makes sense to utilise these properties and to enhance them where possible. Skin assessment should be undertaken daily for the at-risk patient. Where possible the patient and/or carer should be involved in this process. Any alterations in skin status should be recorded immediately; unqualified staff should be alerted to the need to inform the qualified nurses should this arise, as a change in the plan of care may be required.

Skin assessment is important in two ways: it provides baseline data of the initial

Table 5.5   European Pressure Ulcer Advisory Panel guidelines on pressure ulcer prevention.

---

(4) To improve the outcomes for patients at risk of pressure damage through educational programmes

---

- Educational programmes for the prevention of pressure damage should be structured, organised and comprehensive, and made available to all levels of healthcare providers, patients and family or caregivers (C).
- The educational programmes for prevention of pressure damage should include the following items:
    Pathophysiology and risk factors for pressure damage.
    Risk assessment tools and their application.
    Skin assessment.
    Selection and instruction in the use of pressure-redistributing and other devices.
    Development and implementation of individualised programmes of care.
    Principles of positioning to decrease risk of pressure damage.
    Documentation of processes and patient outcome data.
    Clarification of responsibilities for all concerned with this problem.
    Health promotion.
    Development and implementation of guidelines.
- The educational programme should be updated on a regular basis based on the best available evidence. The content of the programme should be modified according to the audience (C).

WATERLOW RISK ASSESSMENT CARD

RING SCORES IN TABLE, ADD TOTAL
SEVERAL SCORES PER CATEGORY CAN BE USED

BUILD/WEIGHT FOR HEIGHT	★	RISK AREAS VISUAL SKIN TYPE	★	SEX AGE	★	SPECIAL RISKS	★
AVERAGE	0	HEALTHY	0	MALE	1	**TISSUE MALNUTRITION:**	★
ABOVE AVERAGE	1	TISSUE PAPER	1	FEMALE	2	eg. TERMINAL CACHEXIA	8
OBESE	2	DRY	1	14 – 49	1	CARDIAC FAILURE	5
BELOW AVERAGE	3	OEDEMATOUS	1	50 – 64	2	PERIPHERAL VASCULAR DISEASE	5
CONTINENCE	★	CLAMMY **T ↑**	1	65 – 74	3	ANAEMIA	2
COMPLETE/ CATHETERISED	0	DISCOLOURED	2	75 – 80	4	SMOKING	1
						NEUROLOGICAL DEFICIT:	★
OCCASION INCONT.	1	BROKEN/SPOT	3	81 +	5	eg DIABETES, CVA	
CATH/INCONTINENT OF FAECES	2	**MOBILITY**	★	**APPETITE**	★	M.S., PARAPLEGIA; MOTOR/SENSORY	4-6
		FULLY	0	AVERAGE	0		
DOUBLY INCONT.	3	RESTLESS/FIDGETY	1	POOR	1	**MAJOR SURGERY/TRAUMA**	★
		APATHETIC	2	N.G. TUBE/		ORTHOPAEDIC – BELOW WAIST, SPINAL	5
		RESTRICTED	3	FLUIDS ONLY	2	ON TABLE > 2 HRS	5
		INERT/TRACTION	4	NBM/ANOREXIC	3	**MEDICATION**	★
		CHAIRBOUND	5			STEROIDS, CYTOTOXICS, ANTI-INFLAMMATORY	4

SCORE:	10+ AT RISK	15+ HIGH RISK	20+ VERY HIGH RISK

© J WATERLOW

Fig. 5.2   The Waterlow Score. Reproduced with permission.

skin status at the beginning of a care episode; and it provides ongoing information on the effectiveness of the prevention plan. Skin assessment involves:

- assessment of the bony prominences, remembering that emaciated patients may develop sores in uncommon areas, e.g. ribs;
- skin status should be identified – dryness, fragility, erythema, areas of maceration are all vulnerable to tissue damage;
- skin colour – dark skin is more difficult to assess for early signs of tissue damage; watch for dryness, cracking or induration.

Traditionally, skin care was provided by rubbing patients' pressure areas, particularly sacrum, buttocks and heels, at regular intervals. A variety of lotions and potions were used. However, this practice has been discredited. Dyson (1978) compared two groups of 100 elderly patients over a six-month period. The control group had their buttocks and sacrum rubbed with soap and water. The other group had their buttocks washed as required only. There was a 38% reduction in pressure sore incidence in the experimental group compared with the control group. A recent review of the literature by Buss *et al.* (1997) considered the effects of massage or rubbing on pressure sore prevention. They concluded that this practice could not be recommended.

When the practice of rubbing was discontinued most nurses developed a reluctance to use any type of cream over the pressure areas. Whilst this is generally appropriate, there may be exceptions in the case of very dry or very moist skin. Emollients should be considered when caring for patients with very dry skin. This can be in the form of emollients in the bath or an emollient cream. Creams should be applied gently to the affected area. If the skin is moist, the source of the moisture should be identified and dealt with if possible. A barrier cream may be needed to protect the skin from the harmful effects of moisture. Frequent cleansing using soap and water for incontinent patients can cause excessive drying of the skin. Dealey and Keogh (1998) found a significant improvement in skin status using a cleanser and barrier cream compared with soap and water in elderly incontinent patients at risk of pressure sore development.

Friction and shear can be reduced by correct positioning, transferring and repositioning techniques. Incorrect positions in either bed or chair can cause patients to slide. Regular moving of patients puts nurses at risk of back injury. One study showed that two nurses on a geriatric ward lifted the equivalent of 2.5 tons in weight in one hour (General, Municipal and Boilermakers Union, 1985). Lifting regulations have been established by a European Community directive indicating the necessity for a policy on manual lifting. In the UK, the Health and Safety Executive produced such a document (1992). All healthcare institutions must have a policy for manual handling and staff should have regular training on correct methods of moving patients. Hoists, slides and other aids for moving patients should be available. The Royal College of Nursing (1996) produced a code of practice which suggests that manual handling should be eliminated in all but exceptional or life-threatening situations. All nurses have a responsibility to take reasonable care for their own safety and for that of patients and colleagues.

If nutritional assessment identifies a patient as having a reduced nutritional status then an appropriate plan of care must be developed. Chapter 2 discusses this in more detail.

As has already been noted, pressure sores may be associated with acute illness. As the general condition of patients improves so their levels of mobility and activity should increase. Some patients may require considerable rehabilitation to optimise their mobility levels. It is important that patients achieve as great a level of mobility and activity as is practical for each individual as immobility has far reaching consequences (see Fig. 2.3, page 31).

(3) Protect against the adverse effects of external mechanical forces: pressure, friction and shear.
Relief of pressure is the main method used in the prevention of pressure sores. This may be achieved by regular repositioning of the patient and the use of pressure-relieving equipment (support systems) when necessary. Patients should be given care appropriate to their specific needs.

For many patients regular repositioning is all that is necessary for pressure sore prevention. Patients should be moved every 2–4 hours depending upon need. The standard method is to turn patients from side to side. Lowthian (1979) designed a 'turning clock' to establish effective positioning. Figure 5.3 shows how it can be used so that a patient can be sitting up at mealtimes and side-lying at others.

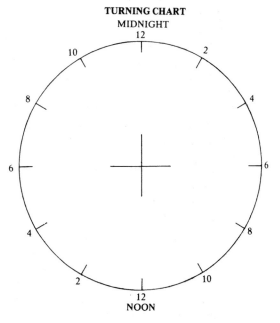

TURNING CHART

INSTRUCTION LIST

MN - 1		7 - 8		2 - 3		9 - 10	
1 - 2		8 - 9		3 - 4		10 - 11	
2 - 3		9 - 10		4 - 5		11 - MN	
3 - 4		10 - 11		5 - 6			
4 - 5		11 - MD		6 - 7			
5 - 6		12 - 1		7 - 8			
6 - 7		1 - 2		8 - 9			

Fig. 5.3 Lothian Turning Clock (from Lothian, 1979).

Oertwich *et al.* (1995) found that even small movements can reduce pressure and increase blood flow over bony prominences. Regular assessment of the pressure areas must be made in order to detect any evidence of excessive pressure; if this occurs other means of pressure relief may be needed.

An alternative to traditional 'turning' of patients is the 30° tilt. This method of positioning patients was developed in a younger disabled unit (Preston, 1988). The patient is placed into a tilted position by the use of pillows (see Fig. 5.4). Once in position, there is no pressure on the sacrum or heels. The interface pressure on the buttock is around 25 mmHg. Colin *et al.* (1996) compared the effect of the 90° lateral position with the 30° tilt and found significant hypoxaemia over the trochanter in the former position but none in the latter.

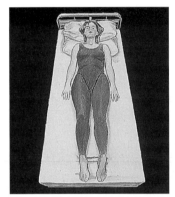

5.4a

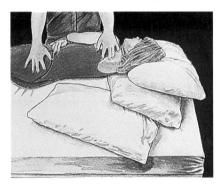

5.4b

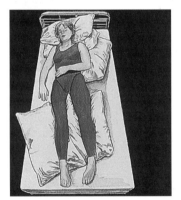

5.4c

Fig. 5.4 The 30 degree tilt. This is a useful method of positioning patients who are difficult to turn or are not able to lie on their side. Patients may be safely left for long periods in this position, but the pressure areas should be carefully monitored to establish an appropriate time for each patient. (a) Place the patient in the centre of the bed with sufficient pillows to support the head and neck. (b) Place a pillow at an angle under one buttock thus tilting the pelvis by 30 degrees. Check with a flattened hand that the sacrum is just clear of the mattress. (c) Place a pillow lengthways under each leg so that the heels are lifted clear of the bed. Reproduced by kind permission of Medical Support Systems Ltd.

Patients can be left for increasingly longer periods without turning, again careful observation must be made of all vulnerable areas. Once patients have become accustomed to using the 30° tilt, they may be left for up to eight hours without turning; not only does this allow an undisturbed night's sleep, but it is of great benefit for use in the community. This method of positioning is not suitable for all patients, but is a useful addition to the skills available for preventing pressure sores.

The standard hospital mattress

Much has been written in recent years about the use of various support systems. Far less time has been spent considering the standard mattress, despite the fact that this is what most patients use. O'Dea (1993) found that 33% of patients with pressure damage were being nursed on a standard hospital mattress. Foam has a finite life-span. The Department of Health recommends that the standard mattress has a life-span of four years. The foam in the mattresses should be at least 130 mm in depth, or it will collapse in a much shorter time. The use of two-way stretch covers gives improved pressure relief, in contrast to Staph Chek covers which increase pressure (Podmore, 1993). The water resistance of the cover can be damaged by the use of alcohol sprays for cleaning, which can also reduce the life of the mattress; cleaning with soap and water is the best method to use.

All hospitals should establish a replacement programme. Mattresses need to be tested annually for grounding and the effectiveness of the cover. Worn out mattresses can then be replaced. The *Effective Health Care Bulletin* (1995) recommends that pressure-relieving foam mattresses should be used for at-risk patients rather than the standard mattress. Many hospitals are replacing worn out standard mattresses with this type of mattress.

Pressure-relieving beds and mattresses

There is an ever increasing range of equipment available for use. They range from overlays to highly sophisticated beds. Some reduce pressure by 'spreading the load' and reducing pressures over bony prominences; others actually relieve pressure, in a variety of ways.

Caution is needed in the purchase of pressure-relieving equipment. Clark and Cullum (1992) found that, despite an increase in the availability of equipment, the prevalence of pressure sores increased over a four-year period. Young (1992) and Bliss and Thomas (1993) have discussed the lack of research into the various pressure-relieving systems available. The *Effective Health Care Bulletin* has examined the evidence regarding the range of product types available and considered that it is not possible to recommend any one product as a 'best buy'. However, they do suggest that high-risk patients are best nursed on a large cell alternating air mattress, a low air loss bed or an air fluidised bed.

Until more conclusive evidence is produced, selection of a support system must depend upon the degree of risk of the patient and individual choice. Dealey (1997) has reviewed the range of support systems and identified their potential use. In many areas, choice is limited according to the availability of equipment. Figure 5.5

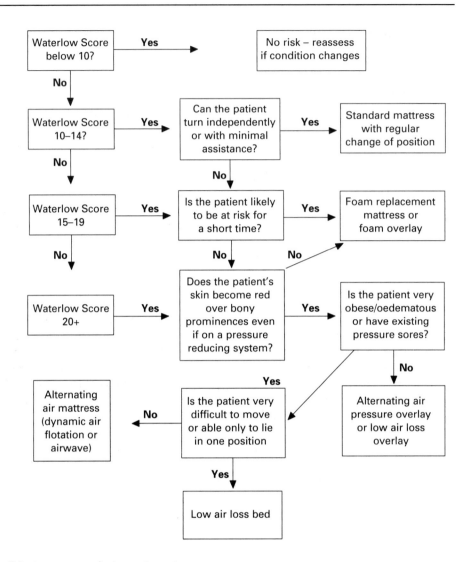

Fig. 5.5 Selecting pressure-relieving equipment.

suggests how equipment can be selected according to the degree of risk of the patient.

Jay (1997) suggested that cost, patient comfort, clinician satisfaction, safety and reliability and logistical considerations need to be taken into consideration as well as efficacy. Some of these factors can be illustrated by considering the water bed. The water bed was widely used during the 1970s. It provided effective pressure reduction. However, it was very unpopular with both nurses and patients. It was extremely heavy and it was sometimes pushed into corners of a ward because of its weight, thus isolating the patient. It was very difficult for individuals to move in the bed or for nurses to move patients. There were also logistical problems with filling and emptying the water and a potential infection hazard if the water was not treated with long-life antimicrobials.

Additions to the bed

Pressure relief can be enhanced by the use of simple measures. The use of bed cradles can lift the weight of the bedclothes off the patient. Back-rests are widely used, but it should be remembered that they cause the patient to slide down the bed, risking damage to the skin by shearing. Strategic placing of pillows can relieve pressure from bony prominences such as heels, the malleoli of the ankles, and the knees. Pads can be applied to the heels or elbows for extra pressure relief. If the patient is out of bed during the day, these pads can be applied at night. Zernikern (1994) compared several devices for heels and found that eggshell foam and foam splints were the most effective.

Chairs

Once ill patients start to be seated out of bed, they are perceived to be 'mobile' and so may be left in the chair for long periods of time without being moved. Many hospital armchairs are in a poor state and fail to give any pressure relief or maintain a good posture (Dealey et al., 1991). Chairs should be checked and replaced or repaired in the same way as mattresses. Many chairs have a reclining back of between 15° and 40° which puts the patient in a semi-reclining posture. This may make it more difficult for the patient to stand. Ideally, a chair should have a recline of not more than 10°, enabling the patient to move more freely. Although cushions may be added to chairs to improve pressure relief, the cushion should not make the chair so high that the patient's feet do not touch the floor. Conventional seating is not suitable for everyone. Some patients have severe seating problems due to contractures, deformity or infirmity; specialised seating must be considered for these people.

Cushions

Most of the research on cushions has been on those for use in wheelchairs. Wheelchairs have a canvas base which Rithalia (1989) found exerted pressures in the region of 226 mmHg. It is essential that a cushion should *always* be used in a wheelchair. For those people who become wheelchair bound because of disability, special assessment should be made to identify the cushion most suited to the specific needs of the patient. Many physiotherapists and occupational therapists have developed specialist skills in assessment. A wide range of cushions is available, made from similar materials to mattresses and overlays.

Other hospital equipment

Vulnerable patients may spend time lying or sitting on very hard surfaces such as operating tables, X-ray tables, trolleys and some types of wheelchair. Very little consideration has been given to the need to provide some sort of pressure relief in these circumstances. Versluysen (1986) undertook a study of 100 consecutive elderly patients admitted with a fractured femur. The interface pressures were measured on the casualty trolleys and operating tables. The casualty trolleys with a 5 cm deep foam mattress showed pressures ranging from 56–60 mmHg at the sacrum and 150–160 mmHg at the heels. The fracture operating table had interface pressures ranging from 75–80 mmHg at the sacrum and 60–120 mmHg at the heels. Bridel (1993b) conducted a small pilot study of 24 patients undergoing surgery. She found an incidence of 12.5% of pressure sores that occurred as a result of damage on the operating table. Hawkins (1997) compared the standard operating table with an air-filled pad and a foam pad for patients undergoing cardiothoracic or major vascular surgery. The results showed a significant reduction in pressure sore incidence in both of the groups using the pads compared with the group lying directly on the operating table.

Every patient at risk of pressure sore development should have an individualised written plan of care. It is important to document all assessments and the care given. This will enable staff to monitor the effectiveness of the plan and to identify any early signs of tissue damage. It should also ensure effective use of equipment as patients may be moved to less sophisticated equipment when they no longer have need of the 'high tech' equipment, or vice versa.

(4) Improve the outcome for patients at risk of pressure damage through educational programmes.
There is little point in developing a policy for pressure sore prevention if no attempt is made to provide relevant education for healthcare professionals and assistants, patients and carers. A number of authors have described the beneficial outcomes of educational programmes. O'Brien *et al.* (1998) found a reduction in the biannual prevalence rate following an educational programme. Danchaivijitr *et al.* (1995) and Regan *et al.* (1995) found a reduction in pressure sore incidence following the introduction of a prevention programme supported by staff education.

Summary

The various aspects of pressure sore prevention can be summarised as follows:

- Assessment: identify those at risk, assess and monitor the skin, especially bony prominences, identify continence problems.
- Plan appropriate preventive measures.
- Evaluate outcomes by maintaining vigilant skin assessment.
- Monitor all support systems, establishing replacement or maintenance programmes where appropriate.
- Ensure staff have an adequate knowledge of causes and prevention of pressure sores.
- Establish a teaching programme for long-term at-risk patients and their carers.
- Monitor outcomes of overall prevention strategies by measuring the prevalence and incidence of pressure sores.

5.2.4 The management of pressure sores

If a pressure sore occurs, preventive measures should still be continued. The precise cause of the sore and the effectiveness of the prevention programme need to be evaluated. Any necessary changes must be made, such as using a different support system or increasing proteins and vitamins in the diet. There are several other factors which need to be considered in the management of pressure sores. They include position of the sore, grading of the sore and its appearance and appropriate selection of wound management products.

The position of pressure sores

Some bony prominences are more prone to pressure sores than others. Lockett (1983) reported on the position of pressure sores found in the survey by David *et al.* (1983). Figure 5.6 shows the range of positions with the percentages found in each. There are some specific aspects of care that need to be considered.

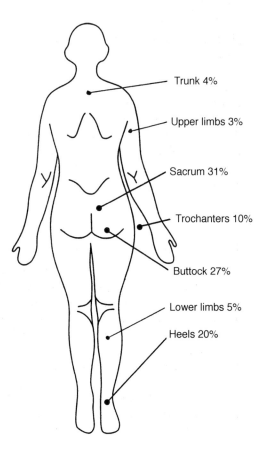

Fig. 5.6 The common position of pressure sores (after Lockett, 1983).

Sacrum: Dressings must be chosen with care, as many tend to ruckle up as the patient moves. Chair sitting must be strictly regulated as to type of chair and length of time seated in it.

Buttocks: As for sacrum.

Heels: Ideally dressings must not be too bulky as this may impede mobility. Dressings may need to be 'tailored' in order to fit correctly around the heel. If footware is being worn, care must be taken to ensure that it is not too tight, or this will exert pressure on the heel. Ensure there is adequate pressure relief when in bed.

Trochanters: Some dressings may ruckle up, so select carefully.

Elbows: Pressure sores are usually caused by friction from moving about the bed. Consider ways of reducing friction – e.g. use of a monkey pole, use of pads or semipermeable film dressings.

Trunk: Sores here are uncommon; try and identify source of pressure and remove or modify it.

Grading of pressure sores

Use of a recognised system of grading pressure sores can be helpful by providing an objective description of a pressure sore. It gives a more accurate picture of the amount of tissue damage than comments such as 'a deep sore'. It should be used in conjunction with other descriptive tools such as measuring or tracing the sore and describing its appearance.

Several methods of grading pressure sores have been put forward. In a review of the relevant literature, Hitch (1995) found ten different grading methods. These systems varied slightly, but in all cases the higher the grade, the deeper the sore. Ideally there should be one recognised grading system. The American National Pressure Ulcer Advisory Panel produced a Consensus Development Statement (National Pressure Ulcer Advisory Panel, 1989) which proposed a grading system that was an amalgam of several commonly used methods of grading. They proposed it should be the start of developing a universally accepted grading system. It is as follows:

Grade I: Non-blanchable erythema of intact skin, heralding skin ulceration.

Grade II: Partial-thickness skin loss involving epidermis and/or dermis. The ulcer is superficial and may be seen as a blister, abrasion or crater.

Grade III: Full-thickness wound involving epidermis, dermis and subcuticular layer. The ulcer presents as a crater with or without undermining.

Grade IV: Extensive destruction involving other tissues such as muscle, tendon or bone.

Figure 5.7 a–d and Plates 15–22 show examples of each of these grades of pressure sore.

Pressure sore appearance

Wound appearance has been discussed in detail in Chapter 3. The same principles can be applied to pressure sores. A pressure sore should be assessed for its appearance as well as its grade. For example, Grades III and IV sores can be necrotic, infected, sloughy or granulating in appearance. Accurate assessment is necessary in order to select a suitable wound management product.

Selection of wound management products

A variety of wound management products can be used when treating pressure sores. The range of wound management products available is discussed in Chapter 4. At present, there is insufficient evidence to determine which dressing is the most appropriate for each grade of pressure sore. It is, of course, entirely possible that such prescriptive wound care would never be appropriate and that a range of products are needed in order to address individual patient need. Many of the studies compare two products and find little or no difference in performance. This may be because there truly is no difference or because the sample size is too small to detect any differences.

Colin *et al.* (1997) compared a film dressing with a thin hydrocolloid dressing for the management of Grade I and II pressure sores ($n = 40$). They found no difference in healing rates, but there was a significantly greater reduction in wound size in the film group compared with the thin hydrocolloid group. Teot *et al.* (1998) compared two thin hydrocolloids on Grade I and II pressure sores and found no differences in outcome ($n = 41$). Both film and thin hydrocolloid dressings would seem to be suitable for these grades of sore.

Several studies have considered appropriate products for Grade II–IV pressure sores. Teot *et al.* (1998a,b) compared a second generation hydrocolloid – a hydrofibre dressing – with a traditional tulle dressing ($n = 62$). The hydrofibre dressing produced a greater healing rate and a greater reduction in wound size. However, these results were not significant. Sopata (1997) compared a gel dressing with an adhesive foam dressing and found no differences in performance between the two ($n = 34$). Seeley *et al.* (1998) found no difference in healing rates in a comparison of a hydrocolloid and an adhesive hydrocellular foam dressing ($n = 40$). A similar study in the UK of the same dressings produced the same results ($n = 61$) (Bale *et al.*, 1997). However, the researchers found a high drop-out rate (26%), unrelated to the dressings, mainly due to patient discharge or death. They proposed that future study designs should include larger patient numbers. Thomas *et al.* (1997) compared a hydropolymer foam dressing with a hydrocolloid dressing ($n = 99$) and found no differences in outcome.

Several researchers have investigated the management of sloughy or necrotic pressure sores. Colin *et al.* (1996) compared a hydrogel with a dextranomer paste ($n = 135$). They found a significant reduction in wound size at 21 days in the hydrogel group. The hydrogel treatment costs were also significantly lower than those of the dextranomer paste. The other studies compared two different hydrogels and found no difference in healing rates (Young *et al.*, 1997; Bale & Crook, 1998; Bale *et al.*, 1998). Hydrogels are effective products for managing sloughy pressure sores, however, there is no evidence to indicate which one out-performs the others.

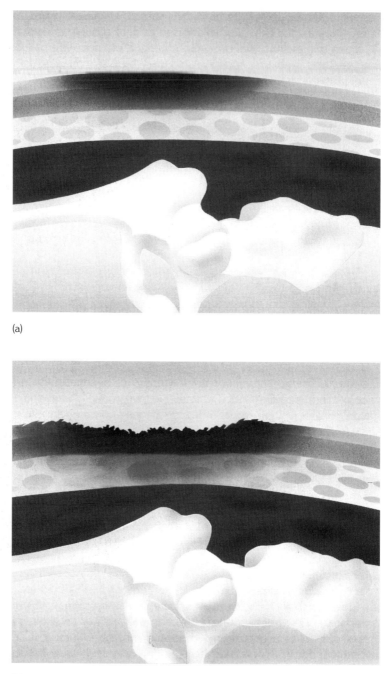

(a)

(b)

Fig. 5.7   Pressure sore grades: (a) Grade I – non-blanchable erythema of intact skin. (b) Grade II – partial-thickness skin loss. (c) Grade III – full-thickness skin loss. (d) Grade IV – full-thickness skin loss with extensive destruction. Reproduced with kind permission of Huntleigh Healthcare Ltd.

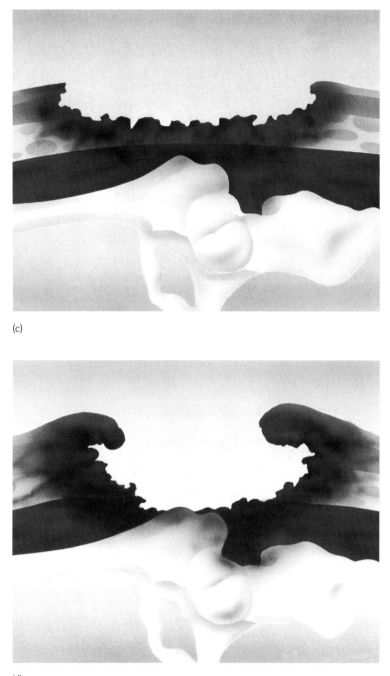

(c)

(d)

Fig. 5.7 *Contd*

The use of plastic surgery

The healing time of a large-cavity pressure sore can be considerably reduced by plastic surgery. However, it is not appropriate for all patients. Their condition may be too poor or the sore may be healing rapidly. Traditionally, reconstructive plastic surgery is most commonly used on patients with spinal cord injury. Khoo and Bailey (1990) have described the principles of reconstructive surgery. They see it to be a series of steps – removal of all necrotic tissue, repeated debridement until healthy granulation tissue is obtained and then closure of the wound using a skin graft or flap. However, there have been reports of recurrence rates of up to 80%. Kierney *et al.* (1998) found that such rates could be reduced by working collaboratively with colleagues in the Department of Physical Medicine and Rehabilitation. In a longitudinal study of 158 patients they found a recurrence rate of 25%. They considered their success was related to improved patient selection combined with a protocol for rehabilitation following surgical repair.

5.3 THE MANAGEMENT OF LEG ULCERS

Leg ulcers are an increasingly common chronic wound and have been recognised for many years. Those following the Hippocratic view that disease was the result of imbalance of the four humours of the body, believed that a leg ulcer allowed the bad humours to leach out. In some areas, this belief still persists – the ulcer lets the bad out and if it heals the person will die. In such circumstances there may be little incentive to conform to treatment.

Until recently there was not much interest amongst doctors in the treatment of this condition. Their views seemed to coincide with that of an eighteenth-century physician who described the care of leg ulcers as 'an unpleasant and inglorious task where much labour must be bestowed and little honour gained' (quoted in Loudon, 1982). Modern developments in wound management have revitalised those caring for patients with leg ulcers.

5.3.1 The epidemiology of leg ulcers

There have been two major surveys carried out within the UK to identify the numbers of people with leg ulcers. The largest was the Lothian and Forth Valley survey in Scotland (Callam *et al.*, 1985). Cornwall *et al.* (1986) surveyed an urban London health district. Surveys have also been carried out in Sweden and Australia (Nelzen *et al.*, 1991; Baker & Stacey, 1994; Ebbeskog *et al.*, 1996). They all found similar results with prevalence rates of 1.3–3.0 per 1000 population which increase to 20 per 1000 in those over 80 years. Dale and Gibson (1986) extrapolated the figures from the Scottish survey and calculated that in the UK there are 440 000 people who could potentially develop ulcers and about 88 000 people with open ulcers. Gilchrist (1989) suggested that the number of people receiving treatment for leg ulcers is about 400 000.

Leg ulcers are predominantly seen to be a condition affecting women. Up to the age of 40, ulcers are fairly equally distributed between the sexes. At the age range of 65–74 years, the female/male ratio is 2.6:1. This increases to a ratio of 10.3:1 over the age of 85 (Dale & Gibson, 1986). This difference is probably, in part, because women live longer than men, but may also be because of the increased risk of deep vein thrombosis during pregnancy.

One of the problematic features of leg ulcers is the length of time they can take to heal and the frequency of recurrence. Baker and Stacey (1994) found that 24% had had their ulcers open for more than a year; 35% for more than five years and 20% of leg ulcer sufferers had had ten or more episodes of ulceration. They also noted that 45% of the leg ulcer population were so immobile as to be house bound.

5.3.2 The cost of leg ulcers

As has already been shown, leg ulcers can be a longstanding and recurrent problem. Inevitably, they are also very expensive to manage. The majority of patients with leg ulcers are cared for in the community and so require home visits or to be taken to clinics. Harkiss (1985) was one of the first to undertake comparative costs of different types of treatment. Although the figures are now dated, it is interesting to note that many of the newer dressings were cheaper to use than more traditional treatments. Gruen et al. (1996) analysed the cost of hospitalisation for leg ulcer patients over a two-year period. They found the patients were admitted for a mean of 44.2 days at a total cost of A$2 750 000. What was even worse was that less than 50% of patients (n = 119) had any documented improvement on discharge. In the UK, Bosanquet (1992) put the cost to the health service at around £400 million a year.

Several centres have established community leg ulcer clinics and costed the outcomes. Simon et al. (1996) compared one community health district having five such clinics with a similar community with no clinics. Both centres had 200–250 patients with leg ulcers. After one year, the community with clinics had reduced expenditure from £409 991 to £253 271 whereas in the other community health district the costs had risen from £556 039 to £673 318. Leg ulcers can be seen as an expensive disease, but potential savings can be made when cost-effective care is instigated.

None of the studies quoted above consider the cost to the patient. Such costs are impossible to quantify. Chase et al. (1997) undertook a qualitative study of 37 ambulant leg ulcer patients which documented the pain suffered by most patients as well as the restrictions it placed on their daily lives, even young men. The study also found that many felt a sense of powerlessness over healing and recurrence rates.

5.3.3 The causes of leg ulcers

There are a variety of causes of leg ulcers. The commonest are venous disease, arterial disease or a combination of the two, generally referred to as mixed ulcers. Another common cause is diabetes. The aetiology and the management of each of these types of ulcer will be considered in turn. Other causes of leg ulceration are infection, neoplasms, inflammatory disease and trauma.

5.3.4 Venous ulcers

Aetiology

Chronic venous insufficiency is the commonest cause of leg ulcers. Callam *et al.* (1985) found that 70% of the ulcers they surveyed were of venous origin. Initially, thrombosis or varicosity causes damage to the valves in the veins of the leg. The deep vein is surrounded by muscle. When the leg is exercised, the calf muscle contracts and squeezes the veins, encouraging the flow of blood along the vein. This is often referred to as the calf muscle pump.

Normally blood flows from the superficial veins to the deep veins via a series of perforator vessels. The valves in the vessels ensure that blood moves from the capillary bed towards the heart (see Fig. 5.8). If some of the valves become damaged then blood can flow in either direction. The backflow of blood towards the capillary bed leads to venous hypertension. As a result, the capillaries become distorted and more permeable. Larger molecules than normal are able to escape into the extravascular space, for example fibrinogen and red blood cells. The haemoglobin is first released from the red blood cells and then broken down causing eczema and a brown staining in the gaiter area. Ultimately there is fibrosis of the underlying tissues giving the leg a 'woody' feeling. This condition is called lipodermatosclerosis. The slightest trauma to the leg and an ulcer will develop. Common examples of trauma are knocking the leg on the corner of a piece of furniture or a fall, injuring the lower leg.

The lymphatic system may also be affected. The lymphatics are responsible for removing protein, fat, cells and excess fluid from the tissues. Ryan (1987) has

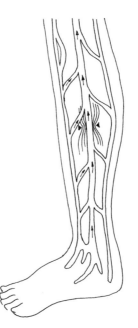

Fig. 5.8   The veins of the leg.

described how the superficial lymphatics in the dermis disappear. This results in waste products accumulating in the tissues which can cause fibrosis and further oedema.

Management

● *Assessment* ●

Full assessment of the patient is essential as many factors can delay the healing of chronic wounds (see Chapter 2). A medical assessment may be necessary to ensure accurate diagnosis. Factors that may need to be particularly considered include nutritional status, mobility, sleeping, smoking, blood and urine testing to screen for anaemia and diabetes, pain, the psychological effects of leg ulceration and the patient's understanding of the disease process. The past medical history may give an indication of any causative factors such as a previous deep vein thrombosis. A history of cardiovascular or rheumatoid disease may be indicative of other problems. A comprehensive assessment of the affected leg must be made, as it is important to rule out arterial disease; the treatments for venous and arterial ulcers are not compatible.

First look at the legs. The characteristic staining of lipodermatosclerosis is usually clearly seen in the gaiter area. Ankle flare may also be present. This is distension of the network of small veins situated just below the medial malleolus. Oedema may be present, but can also be found in arterial ulceration. Theoretically, the leg and foot should feel warm to touch, but if the weather is cold this may not be the case. The skin surrounding the ulcer may be fragile and eczematous.

Typically, venous ulcers are found on or near the medial malleolus. They tend to be shallow and develop slowly over a period of time. They are frequently painful. Hofman *et al.* (1997) interviewed 94 patients with venous ulcers and found that 64% had severe pain, 38.3% had continuous pain and 63.8% were woken by pain. It should also be noted that pain will be increased if there is any infection in the ulcer. The appearance of the ulcer should be assessed as in Chapter 3. Many venous ulcers have a heavy exudate. Plate 23 shows a typical venous ulcer with staining in the gaiter area.

Differential diagnosis between venous and arterial ulcers can be made by assessing the blood supply to the leg. This is best achieved by means of Doppler ultrasonography. This procedure should be undertaken by staff who have received training so to do. Doppler ultrasonography is used to compare the blood pressure in the lower leg to the brachial pressure. It is usually presented in the form of a ratio, the ankle/brachial pressure index (ABPI), which is calculated by the following formula:

$$\frac{\text{Ankle systolic pressure}}{\text{Brachial systolic pressure}} = \text{Ankle/brachial pressure index}$$

An ABPI of 0.9 or above indicates a normal arterial supply to the leg. If it is below 0.9 then some ischaemia is present. Compression therapy should not be used if the

ABPI is below 0.8. If there is any doubt about the presence of arterial disease, further medical opinion should be sought.

● *Planning* ●

There are three aspects to the management of venous ulcers: improving the drainage of the leg; skin care; and the use of appropriate wound management products. Any one of these alone will not be truly effective without the others.

The drainage of the legs can be improved in several ways: exercise, compression and elevation. The use of exercise stimulates the calf muscle pump, promoting drainage. Allen (1983) recommends that patients should walk as much as they are able and, if standing still, move from one foot to the other. He also suggests that frequent ankle exercises should be performed when sitting. Obviously exercise should be tailored to the abilities of the patient. Regular encouragement will be needed to ensure patients persist with their exercises.

Compression works with exercise to aid drainage from the superficial veins. It should be graduated so that there is a higher pressure at the ankle than at the calf. It can be achieved by the use of either bandages or stockings. Bandages are probably easiest to use in the early stages when the dressings may be rather bulky. Some remain in place day and night whereas others may be removed at night. When applying bandages it is best done before the patient rises, when the leg has the least amount of oedema.

Thomas (1990) has categorised compression bandages into four groups:

● Light compression giving 14–17 mmHg at the ankle.
● Moderate compression giving 18–24 mmHg at the ankle.
● High compression giving 25–35 mmHg at the ankle.
● Extra high compression giving 60 mmHg at the ankle.

The level of compression needed for venous ulceration is around 40 mmHg, (Stemmer, 1969). Therefore, the high compression bandages should be suitable. However, these pressures are dependent on the size of the limb. A large limb, swollen with oedema, would require a higher compression bandage than a thinner limb in order to achieve an adequate level of compression. There is also considerable skill in applying a compression bandage correctly and it is regrettable that bandaging is often not included in the curriculum for nurse training. Logan *et al.* (1992) found inconsistency in application amongst inexperienced bandagers when compared with more experienced staff. Magazinovic *et al.* (1993) found registered nurses lacked understanding of the principles of bandaging. The manufacturer's instructions should always be followed when applying any bandage. The commonest method is to apply the bandage in a spiral, as shown in Fig. 5.9.

A systematic review of clinical trials of compression bandaging found that multilayer bandage systems were the most effective method of achieving compression (Fletcher *et al.*, 1997). Multilayer systems usually comprise three or four layers. They consist of orthopaedic padding, crepe, elastic bandage and a cohesive layer (four layer) or orthopaedic padding, crepe and high compression bandage (three layer). The benefit of the orthopaedic padding is that it helps to absorb excess

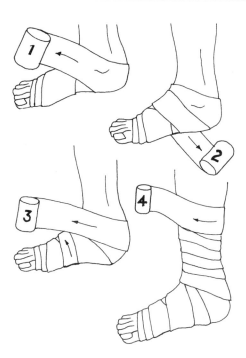

Fig. 5.9 Application of a spiral bandage.

exudate and can provide extra padding over bony prominences. In mainland Europe the short-stretch bandage is widely used. This bandage is applied in a combination of figures of eight and spirals which achieve a multilayer effect.

Tubular bandages may also be used to provide compression. The straight variety do not give appropriate compression as pressure is higher at the calf than the ankle. There is a shaped tubular bandage which can be most useful as it is relatively easy to apply. This type of compression may be the easiest to pull on for someone with arthritic hands. It is more effective to use two layers of bandage. It must be recognised that the tubular bandage does not provide the level of compression provided by the multilayer systems. However, for those patients who cannot tolerate high compression it may be a viable alternative.

Below-knee compression stockings are widely used as the ulcer improves, and after healing. Some manufacturers also produce compression socks for men which look like ordinary socks. For many patients, socks and stockings are easier to apply than bandages. Jones and Nelson (1998) have reviewed the use of compression stockings. The British Standards Institute has specified three classes of stockings which are available on prescription. The three classes provide different ranges of compression at the ankle:

- Class I has pressures of 14–18 mmHg.
- Class II has pressures of 18–24 mmHg.
- Class III has pressures of 25–35 mmHg.

It is very important that the patient should be correctly fitted for a stocking. Class II may be appropriate for many patients. If a Class III stocking is required, but the patient is unable or unwilling to pull it on, it may be better to use two layers of Class I stockings. Fentem (1986) has shown that this would provide the same level of compression. Compliance is essential for this form of treatment. Mayberry et al. (1991) were able to achieve 97% healing with patients who were compliant and wore their compression stockings, but only 55% healing with those who were noncompliant.

Franks et al. (1995) randomly allocated 166 patients to one of two types of compression stockings following healing of their ulcers. There was no significant difference in results between the two groups. The overall recurrence rate was 26% at 12 months despite a compliance rate of 82.5%. The researchers also found that 15% could not put on their stockings at all and a further 26% had great difficulty in doing so. Furthermore, 30% showed signs of skin irritation under their stockings after one week.

Patients are usually prescribed two pairs of stockings so that they have 'one to wash and one to wear'. This will get the maximum wear out of the stocking. Dale and Gibson (1990) suggest that the stockings should be washed by hand after each wearing. Thus, the stocking should have a life-span of three to four months before being replaced.

Another method of applying compression which can be used, particularly if oedema is present, is pneumatic compression. It may be applied once or twice a day for periods of up to an hour. Initially the time should be shorter and gradually increased. Although this may be a useful form of treatment, it is difficult in the community where there is limited access to such equipment. The use of pneumatic compression should be seen as an addition to the treatment regime rather than an alternative. Mulder et al. (1990) studied the use of sequential pneumatic compression in ten patients with chronic venous ulcers. It was used in addition to paste bandages and compression bandages. They found that pneumatic compression significantly reduced healing time.

Elevation of the legs will also help as it allows gravity to aid venous return. However, many people tend to place their feet on a low stool which is of no benefit whatsoever. To be effective the feet should be higher than the heart. If there is an acute exacerbation of the ulcer with oedema and heavy exudate, it may be worthwhile admitting the patient to hospital for a short period of bedrest. Bedrest with elevation of the foot of the bed can significantly reduce oedema and improve venous return. It should not be considered as a long-term measure because the ulcer will merely break down again once the patient is up and about. It may also seriously affect the mobility of older patients.

A more practical method is to raise the foot of the bed with bricks or blocks of wood at home so that the patient's legs are elevated at night time. The patient should be encouraged to elevate the legs for periods during the day. Ryan (1987) describes the use of a 'Legs up' chart (Fig. 5.10) to encourage patients to elevate their legs for a total of at least two hours during the day, the intention being to actively involve patients in their own care.

Management of the ulcer involves cleansing and a suitable topical application. Consideration must be given to the presence of eczema, scaling on the legs around the ulcer, any allergies to treatment and wound infection.

HELPING TO HEAL YOUR LEG ULCER.

If you have a venous leg ulcer, you can contribute immensely to the rate at which it heals simply by keeping your feet up every day as part of your routine.

By sitting for a short time each day in a comfortable 'legs up' position, as illustrated below, you can help your nurse to heal the wound.

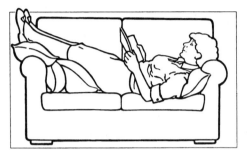

Simply record on the chart overleaf the number of hours that you have spent in the 'legs up' position each day. When the chart is full, give it back to your nurse.

The nurse will then be able to tell you if you are resting your legs enough to ensure a speedy recovery.

PATIENT 'LEGS UP' RECORD CHART

NAME   DATE

Enter in each square below the number of hours you have rested with your legs up.

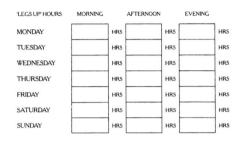

'LEGS UP' HOURS	MORNING	AFTERNOON	EVENING
MONDAY	HRS	HRS	HRS
TUESDAY	HRS	HRS	HRS
WEDNESDAY	HRS	HRS	HRS
THURSDAY	HRS	HRS	HRS
FRIDAY	HRS	HRS	HRS
SATURDAY	HRS	HRS	HRS
SUNDAY	HRS	HRS	HRS

REMEMBER TO GIVE BACK THE COMPLETED CHART TO YOUR NURSE.

Fig. 5.10 'Legs up' chart. From: Ryan, T.J. (1987) *The Management of Leg Ulcers*, 2nd edn. Oxford University Press, Oxford. Reproduced by courtesy of Prof. T.J. Ryan.

Cleansing is an important factor as many patients may have been told in the past that they must never get their ulcer wet. As a result they may not have had a bath for years. Foot baths are very useful as they allow the patient the opportunity to give the affected leg a good soak. Plain tap water is suitable for most patients. Attention needs to be paid to the adequate cleansing of the foot bath after use. If the patient has weeping eczema, a potassium permanganate 0.01% solution can be used. It has a slightly astringent effect.

Paste bandages are widely used in the treatment of leg ulcers. They are cotton bandages impregnated with different types of paste according to the manufacturer. They are soothing to sore, eczematous legs and will also lift off some of the scales that tend to form around the ulcer. Paste bandages do not provide compression, but they enhance the effect of the compression bandages used over the top. Paste bandages have to be applied in such a way as to allow for any swelling of the leg. This may be achieved by making a pleat on each turn at the front of the leg. An alternative method is to overlap each turn and cut the bandage. Paste bandages can be left in place for up to a week.

When taking an initial history, any reported allergies should be noted. Many long-term leg ulcer sufferers develop allergies to their treatment. Cameron (1998) has reviewed the problems of allergic contact dermatitis or contact sensitivity.

Substances which have been found to cause sensitivities include lanolin, neomycin, framycetin, emulsifiers such as cetyl alcohol, rubber, parabens and colophony. Cameron recommends avoiding the use of any products containing potential irritants. Bland emollients such as a 50/50 mixture of soft white paraffin and liquid paraffin ('50/50') should be applied following cleansing of the leg. This can be massaged gently into the skin, helping to lift the skin scales which rapidly build up on the leg. Plate 24 demonstrates the effectiveness of this type of emollient; here '50/50' has been applied to the foot and the skin is clear of scales, unlike the ankle which is still covered in scales.

As with any wound, bacteria colonise the ulcer surface. This has been previously discussed in Chapter 3. If there is any indication of infection and/or cellulitis, medical opinion should be requested. One particular pathogenic organism which gives cause for concern in leg ulcers is β-haemolytic *Streptococcus*. Schraibman (1987) described the relationship between the organism and giant ulcers which did not readily respond to treatment. He suggests systemic antibiotics to eliminate the bacteria, followed by skin grafting.

Management of the ulcer depends on the assessment and the factors previously discussed. Selection of suitable dressings is discussed in Chapter 4. Recently there have been several clinical trials of modern products on leg ulcers which have shown the effectiveness of their use. Overall, there is insufficient evidence to recommend one product over another. Alginates, beads, hydrocolloids and hydrogels may be particularly effective. It should be remembered that although the ulcer may be new to the nurse, the patient may have lived with it for some time. There may be a credibility gap as the patient starts yet another course of treatment which it is stated, will definitely resolve the problem. Effective communication is essential to ensure that the patient understands and is prepared to comply with treatment.

● *Evaluation* ●

Regular assessment of the ulcer may be done by the use of tracings or photographs. They are essential to monitor the progress of the ulcer. If there appears to be no improvement over a period of 2–3 months the ulcer should be re-assessed and any ischaemia or infection ruled out. Patient assessment will identify any relevant factors such as loss of appetite. Skin care should be maintained as the skin is likely to remain scaly.

Patients still need to be seen regularly once the ulcer is healed in order to provide encouragement and to ensure that the preventive care is understood. They should also be given information on how to get further help if the ulcer recurs. The sooner that appropriate care can be given, the sooner the ulcer will heal. Prevention is obviously better than cure. If lipodermatosclerosis is observed, the person should be encouraged to wear compression stockings. Patient education is essential in order for there to be full understanding of the potential hazard of ulceration. Screening programmes – where blood pressure, urine and other similar checks are made – would be an ideal opportunity to check for evidence of lipodermatosclerosis.

5.3.5 Arterial ulcers

Aetiology

Arterial ulcers are the result of inadequate tissue perfusion to the feet or legs, due to complete or partial blockage of the arterial supply to the legs; the underlying condition is often referred to as peripheral vascular disease. This is a general term to encompass disease which reduces the blood supply to the periphery. The commonest disease is arteriosclerosis where the artery walls become thickened. It is usually found in combination with atherosclerosis – the formation of plaques on the inner lining of the vessels. The lumen of the vessels gradually narrows causing ischaemia in the surrounding tissue, ultimately resulting in necrosis. This type of arterial insufficiency is most commonly found in men over the age of 50.

Buerger's disease is another type of disease affecting the peripheral arteries. Inflammation of the vessels results in thrombus formation and occlusion of the vessels. It is associated with heavy smoking and is found most commonly in men between 20 and 35 years old. Ulceration associated with necrosis and gangrene may develop.

Management

• *Assessment* •

Assessment of the patient may reveal pain particularly associated with walking which is relieved by resting – known as intermittent claudication. Pain may also occur at night when the patient is in bed and can be relieved by hanging the legs down. Past medical history may reveal known peripheral vascular disease or arterial surgery. A past or present history of smoking should also be noted.

When the legs are examined they may feel cold to touch and have a shiny, hairless appearance. The toe nails may be thickened and opaque. The legs become white when elevated and a reddish/blue colour when dependent. Pedal pulses are diminished or absent. Doppler ultrasonography will reveal the presence of ischaemia with an ABPI below 0.9. If the patient has intermittent claudication, the ABPI is likely to be between 0.5 and 0.9. If it is below 0.5, rest pain is also likely to be present. The patient should be referred to a vascular surgeon.

Ulcers may occur anywhere on the leg or foot but are most commonly found on the foot; they have a punched out appearance and may be deep, involving muscles or tendons. Necrosis is often present and there is far less exudate than in venous leg ulcers, see Plate 25. Table 5.6 compares venous and arterial ulcers (Dealey, 1991b).

• *Planning* •

Arterial ulcers are notoriously difficult to heal and there is considerable risk of the onset of worsening gangrene and even septicaemia. Amputation of the limb may be the only solution for some. Arterial surgery to improve the blood supply may be necessary before an ulcer will heal. Early referral for reconstructive surgery is ideal.

Table 5.6 A comparison of venous and arterial ulcers.

Sign/symptom	Venous ulcer	Arterial ulcer
Site:	On/near medial malleolus	May be on toes, foot, heel of lateral aspect of leg
Development:	Develops slowly	Develops rapidly
Appearance of ulcer:	Shallow margin; deep tissue not affected	Often deep with involvement of tendons or muscles
Appearance of leg:	Brown, varicose staining and eczema, warm to touch	Shiny skin, cold to touch, white on elevation, may become blue when dependent
Oedema:	Present – usually worse at end of day	Only present if patient immobile – statis oedema
Pain:	Pain varies	Very painful – worse at night. Relieved by hanging leg over side of bed
Medical history:	DVT, phlebitis, varicose veins	Peripheral vascular disease, ischaemic heart disease, diabetes mellitus

Adapted from Dealey, C. (1991b).

Ray *et al.* (1995) found that percutaneous transluminal angioplasty was effective in promoting healing in all those with ulcers in their study ($n = 14$).

If a patient has severe resting pain, good pain control is an essential part of the management. The patient should also be encouraged to give up smoking as failure to do so will further compromise the blood supply to the leg. Gentle exercise will help to encourage the development of a collateral supply to the limb, thus improving tissue perfusion. The limbs should be kept warm as cold may precipitate pain.

The major aim of ulcer management is to remove necrotic tissue and to prevent infection. Selection of appropriate wound management products depends on the ulcer appearance, the amount of exudate and the position of the ulcer (see Chapter 4). The dressing needs to be effectively retained and yet not be so bulky as to restrict mobility unduly. Areas such as the toes are not at all easy to dress.

Bandages are often needed to hold the dressing in place. Compression bandages should not be used on arterial ulcers. Comfortable retention bandages such as cotton conforming bandages are suitable. Lightweight tubular bandages can be very useful, particularly on toes. It is important to ensure that, whatever bandage is used, it does not constrict the blood supply.

● *Evaluation* ●

The progress of both the patient and the ulcer should be evaluated. The effectiveness of pain control can be ascertained using a pain ruler (see Section 2.2.2). When monitoring the progress of the ulcer, attention should be paid to any indications of infection.

5.3.6 Ulcers of mixed aetiology

Some patients will have both an arterial and a venous component to their ulcer. It is important to define the predominant factor, so that appropriate treatment may be given.

Management

● *Assessment* ●

Doppler ultrasonography and assessment of the leg will provide an indication of the mixed aetiology. A full assessment in a vascular laboratory may be of benefit.

● *Planning* ●

If the main factor is venous, moderate graduated compression should be worn during the day. The degree of compression should be based on patient tolerance. Most patients will need to remove the compression garment at night when elevation of the legs is likely to increase ischaemic pain. When arterial disease predominates, compression may be impractical. However, exercise and short periods of limb elevation can be encouraged, within the limits of patient toleration.

● *Evaluation* ●

If healing is very slow, further advice from a vascular surgeon should be obtained.

5.3.7 Diabetic ulcers

Ulceration of the foot is a serious complication of diabetes mellitus affecting about 15% of people with diabetes. Connor (1997) has calculated that in England alone diabetic foot ulcers lead to 4800 amputations annually, of which half are major amputations. Connor further calculated that the cost of this surgery and the concomitant treatment was £38.06 million at 1996 prices. The Department of Health is a signatory to the St Vincent Declaration of 1989 (Conference Report, 1990) which set the target to reduce lower limb amputations by 50% over five years. It is widely accepted that improved foot care and increased vascular investigations and reconstructive surgery are necessary to achieve this. Connor estimated that if adequate prophylactic care was introduced to meet the 50% target there would be potential savings of £19 million a year.

Aetiology

The underlying causes of diabetic ulcers are peripheral neuropathy and peripheral vascular disease. Infection is an ever-present risk for the diabetic patient and can exacerbate the development of ulceration and increase the risk of amputation.

Peripheral neuropathy affects the peripheral sensory, motor and autonomic nerves of the leg. This has a two-fold effect of causing a loss of sensation and compromising the biomechanics of the foot. Muscle atrophy in the foot, particularly over the arch of the foot causes a transfer of body weight and reactive callus formation on the plantar surface. Ultimately, deformities of the foot, such as claw toes or Charcot foot, may occur along with alterations in gait. Walters *et al.* (1993) found foot ulceration was significantly associated with foot deformity. Poorly fitting shoes or a foreign body within the shoe can cause undetected injury resulting in ulcer formation. The patient may be completely unaware of the ulcer for some time.

Vascular disease in diabetic patients primarily affects the smaller arterioles within the foot. Intermittent claudication is unlikely as larger arteries are not usually occluded. Diabetic vascular disease is exacerbated by smoking. Gangrene of the toes can be caused by thrombosis in the artery supplying the affected digit. Pressure from poorly fitting shoes is the commonest cause of ischaemic ulceration.

Microvascular dilatation plays a significant role in the healing of minor wounds. The ability of these vessels to dilate can be measured by using a laser Doppler to test the response to heat. A study by Sandeman *et al.* (1991) considered the ability to respond to heat by vasodilation in insulin-dependent (ID) diabetic patients, non insulin-dependent (NID) diabetic patients and a control group of healthy individuals. A significantly worse response was found in the NID diabetic patients than in the other two groups.

Prevention

Given the grave implications of ulceration, prevention is very important. This can be achieved by patient education and adequate monitoring of the patient by the healthcare team. A multicentre study (Masson *et al.*, 1989) found that only 29% of 51 diabetic patients with new foot ulcers had previously considered that they were at risk of developing ulcers. Although many of the patients in the study were aware of the potential for foot problems, they did not consider themselves to be vulnerable. Litchfield and Ramkissoon (1996) monitored the outcome of providing an educational foot care video for diabetic patients. They found that, although most patients were aware of the need for good foot care, there was a lack of compliance with the recommended care. Healthcare professionals have a responsibility to provide education for the patients in their care, but if patients choose not to accept this advice, it is ultimately their decision. Foster (1997) proposed that a psychologist should be a member of the foot care team in order to help address some of the issues that may lead patients to fail to comply with care and to support patients in coping with the implications of their disease.

Clinical guidelines for the management of diabetic foot disease have been produced in Scotland (Scottish Intercollegiate Guidelines Network [SIGN], 1997). They propose that diabetic patients should be placed in one of three risk categories:

Level 1   No clinical evidence of neuropathy or peripheral vascular disease.
Level 2   Patients with 'at risk' feet (see Table 5.7).
Level 3   Patients with ulceration or gangrene with high risk of amputation.

Table 5.7   Factors increasing the risk of foot ulceration in diabetic patients.

- Previous ulceration
- Neuropathy
- Peripheral vascular disease
- Callus
- Foot deformity
- Poor vision
- Physical disability
- Elderly
- Living alone

All diabetic patients should have annual screening to monitor any changes in risk level (SIGN, 1997). This should include assessment for neuropathy and of the peripheral circulation. It should be noted that Doppler ultrasound assessments may be misleading as calcification of the small vessels may produce an abnormally high false reading. Assessment of the skin will identify any callus formation, fissures or blisters. The foot should also be assessed for any deformity such as claw toes. Patients falling into the Level 1 category should be given general foot care education.

Once patients have been identified as being at risk, then they should be made aware of this and of their responsibilities for prevention of foot problems. Feet should be washed daily and dried carefully. They should be inspected for any red areas, swelling or cracked or broken skin. Toe nails should be cut straight across. Socks should be changed daily and not wrinkle. Shoes should be well fitting. They should be checked before wearing for any foreign bodies. New shoes should be properly fitted and feet carefully observed for signs of rubbing. The patient should not wear sandals or go barefoot. Those with poor vision may need assistance. Those who smoke should stop.

At each attendance at the diabetic clinic, the patient should have a full foot check. This may involve the doctor, diabetic nurse specialist and chiropodist/podiatrist. Treatment of callus formation and management of any fungal infections are usually carried out by the chiropodist/podiatrist. If the patient has any deformity of the feet it may be helpful for the orthotist to assess for suitable footwear. If the patient has other pathology requiring treatment, other health professionals should be vigilant in identifying any potential foot problems.

Management

● *Assessment* ●

When assessing the patient there may be an indication of the type of ulcer. A history of pain associated with the ulcer, for example, almost certainly indicates ischaemia. Deformities of gait are indicative of neuropathy. Assessment of the diabetic state is important because of the increased risk of infection in the presence of hyperglycaemia.

Assessment of the leg and foot will provide objective evidence of the presence of either ischaemia or neuropathy or both. Table 5.8 indicates the differences between the two types of ulcers. However, both pathologies may be present in many patients. This mixed aetiology has been found in 40% of patients seen at a foot hospital (Young & Boulton, 1991). One aspect of assessment is to identify the precipitating factor. Careful assessment of footwear and the precise position of the ulcer can provide clues. It is essential to identify the cause of the ulcer, otherwise further ulceration may occur.

Neuropathic ulcers may be surrounded by callus and have a punched out appearance (see Plate 26). Ischaemic ulcers are usually covered by necrotic tissue.

Table 5.8   A comparison of neuropathic and ischaemic foot ulcers in the diabetic patient.

Sign/symptom	Neuropathic ulcer	Ischaemic ulcer
Deformity of the foot:	Present as claw toe, hammer toe, Charcot foot or other	Not present
Skin temperature of foot:	Warm	Cold
Colour of foot:	Normal	White when elevated or cyanotic
Toe nails:	Atrophic	Atrophic
Pedal pulses:	Present	ABPI below 0.9 (false high readings if small vessels calcified)
Pain:	None	Present, relieved by hanging legs down
Callus formation:	Present, especially on plantar surface	Not present
Ulcer site:	Commonly on plantar surface of foot	Commonly on toes and the edges of the foot

Neither type of ulcer generally has much exudate. The ulcer should be carefully observed for any indication of infection.

Wagner (1981) devised a scale for assessing diabetic ulcers:

Grade 0 At risk foot.
Grade 1 Superficial ulcer, not clinically infected.
Grade 2 Deeper ulcer, often infected, no osteomyelitis.
Grade 3 Deeper ulcer, abscess formation, osteomyelitis.
Grade 4 Localised gangrene (toe, forefoot or heel).
Grade 5 Gangrene of whole foot.

Ulcers graded 0–3 tend to be predominantly neuropathic, whereas in those graded 4 or 5 ischaemia is the main factor.

● *Planning* ●

Adequate control of the diabetic state is the primary goal when managing patients with foot ulceration. Pain control may also be necessary. Management of the ulcer depends on the causative factors. On the whole, neuropathic ulcers should be referred to the chiropodist/podiatrist as the callus needs to be removed before the ulcer can heal. Pressure must also be removed from the ulcer and this can be achieved by felt inserts, contact casting or even the use of crutches. Ischaemic ulcers may be resistant to treatment. Necrotic tissue must be debrided by use of appropriate wound management products. Any infection should be treated with systemic antibiotics and the application of suitable dressings (see Section 4.6). Compression bandages should not be used, but, if necessary, a simple retention bandage can be used to hold the dressing in place. Dermagraft® has been found to be effective in treating diabetic foot ulcers (Grey *et al.*, 1998). Further research on the effectiveness of this product is still taking place.

● *Evaluation* ●

Measurement of the ulcer by tracing may not provide adequate information as the surface area may not appear to alter greatly. A photographic record may be of more value. Careful assessment for any indication of infection should be made at each dressing change. Failure to respond to treatment can result in osteomyelitis. Surgical treatment is then necessary to eradicate the infection. Patients with ischaemic ulcers should be referred for a vascular consultation. Once the ulcer is healed, preventive measures need to be instigated.

5.3.8 Conclusions

Ulceration of the leg can cause untold suffering to the individual. It is important to remember that many of the sufferers are elderly and that they may have other underlying problems which can affect their healing potential. In their report of a pilot leg ulcer clinic, Bliss and Schofield (1993) describe the many problems they found in 26 patients with a mean age of 80 years. When caring for patients with leg ulcers, nurses should be aware of current best practice. However, they may have to be pragmatic in planning individual care and accept that best practice may not always be achievable. Leg ulcer care is very much the 'art of the possible'.

5.4 THE MANAGEMENT OF FUNGATING WOUNDS

Malignant fungating wounds are particularly difficult wounds to manage. They are distressing for both the sufferer and the nurse. A major problem is that there has been very little research into the management of this type of lesion. Most information seems to be anecdotal and nurses provide care based on previous experience or trial and error. Many of the patients with fungating wounds are cared for in the community. Although undoubtedly their nurses devote much time to caring for them, there is a need for research to be undertaken to improve the quality of life of these patients.

A postal survey (Thomas, 1992) has provided information about current practice in radiotherapy centres across the UK. Thomas noted that several respondents commented on the lack of published data and the generally unscientific approach to the management of fungating wounds. Little has changed in the years since the survey was undertaken. Indeed, in a review of fungating wound management, Grocott (1995) considered that the problems raised by Sims and Fitzgerald (1985) had still to be resolved.

5.4.1 Aetiology

Fungating lesions occur when a cancerous mass invades the epithelium, thus ulcerating through to the body surface. It most commonly occurs with cancer of the breast (Sims & Fitzgerald, 1985). However it may also be found in cancers of the skin, vulva and bladder. Fungating wounds do not develop only at the site of the primary tumour; if the nodes of the groin or axilla are affected, ulceration may occur. Rosen (1980) suggests that almost any cancer may develop secondary deposits in the skin, which can then ulcerate.

Fungating lesions are often associated with neglect. That is, the patient delays seeking medical help. This is commonly seen in patients with breast cancers. A typical example is a lady who 'ignored' her breast lump for several years and only when her family noticed the offensive odour did she seek help.

5.4.2 Incidence

Little information seems to be available on this aspect of fungating wounds. Ivetic and Lyne (1990) have reviewed the literature and found no significant research. There seems to be some evidence that fungating lesions of the breast are less common than they once were, but it is not conclusive. Thomas's survey (1992) found that breast lesions were most commonly seen, followed by head and neck lesions. However, the survey did not attempt to assess incidence.

5.4.3 The management of fungating wounds

Management of the patient

This is a vital part of the management of these wounds. Many factors within the patient can affect the progress of the wound. Chapter 2 discusses patient care in greater detail. Factors that need to be considered are:

Communication   patients may find it too difficult to discuss their condition and its implications. Pain may also be a problem that needs to be addressed.

Eating and drinking   nutritional status may be affected by the disease process or by treatment such as radiotherapy or chemotherapy.

Elimination   poor nutrition may result in constipation. Some analgesia may also have the same effect. Ultimately, constipation will cause loss of appetite.

Mobility   poor mobility may affect the patient's ability to be self-caring.

Expressing sexuality   most patients are greatly distressed by their altered body image.

Sleeping   this may be disturbed because of anxiety and/or pain.

Dying   the prognosis for these patients is generally poor. Patients and their family are likely to need help in coming to terms with this.

Medical intervention   radiotherapy treatment may be given to reduce the size of the lesions and resolve some of the symptoms.

Psychological assessment   the patient may show signs of grief, fear or loss of self-respect. Some patients may talk of feeling 'unclean' or show embarrassment, especially when the wound is being dressed. Fitzgerald (Sims & Fitzgerald, 1985) describes how one lady talked of herself as 'leprous' and felt ashamed of her wound because it must be her fault. Patients who feel like that may not want others to dress their wound because they, the patients, believe that the wound would horrify them.

Spiritual assessment   the patient may question the meaning of life or express feelings of guilt and see the lesion as a form of punishment.

Management of the wound

Chapter 3 covers the general principles of wound management. This section will address the specific problems related to fungating wounds.

● *Assessment* ●

When assessing the wound the following need to be considered:

(1) Fungating lesions are often necrotic, sloughy or infected.
(2) There are usually copious amounts of exudate, which may have an offensive odour.
(3) Many of these wounds become malodorous as a result of bacterial invasion. It causes distress to the patient, relatives and visitors, and may be very difficult to control.
(4) The position of the wound obviously depends on the type of cancer. However, it may spread along the trunk or limbs, sometimes in the form of isolated nodules. Plate 27 shows a fungating lesion which has spread under the axilla to

the patient's back. Applying a dressing to protect such a widespread lesion can be very difficult and requires considerable nursing skill.

(5) Capillary bleeding may occur as the cancer increases in size and erodes blood vessels, and may be sufficiently heavy or frequent to cause anaemia. Removal of the old dressing must be done with great care in order to avoid loosening any clots.

(6) Lymphoedema may be present with cancers of the breast, cervix or vulva. This is a chronic swelling of the adjacent limb(s) due to a failure of lymph drainage, and may be associated with loss of function of the affected limb. Logan (1995) reviewed studies of the prevalence of lymphoedema associated with breast cancer and reported that it affects around 25–28% of patients. A small study by Werngren-Elgstrom and Lidman (1994) of patients with cancer of the cervix found that 40% had some limb swelling and 22% of women had symptoms of lymphoedema.

• *Planning* •

It is essential to identify patient problems rather than nurse problems. Although in many instances they may be the same, they are not always. The following is an extreme example encountered by the author.

> Mrs B. was admitted to hospital with a severely swollen leg due to lymphoedema. The ulceration in her groin was relatively small, but there was an ulcer on her leg which constantly poured lymph fluid. Despite being dressed by the district nurses three times a day, her leg was constantly wet and very painful. Initially, the problem of a painful wound was addressed by applying an extra absorbent hydrocolloid dressing. Within 48 hours, the pain had gone and Mrs B. looked a different person. The dressing was being changed daily. The nursing staff decided that the next problem to tackle was the lymphoedema, which would have the effect of reducing the fluid flowing from her leg. When Mrs B. was approached, she categorically said she was not interested. She wanted to go home as she had 'things to sort out' and she knew the district nurses would come and change her dressing when she needed them to do so. Mrs B. went home having had her problem resolved.

Once the specific problems have been identified, the treatment options have to be planned in the light of the patient's condition. If the expected outcome is very poor, then totally palliative care with the minimum need to dress the wound must be the treatment of choice. For others, a more aggressive approach can be used. A course of radiotherapy may be prescribed to help reduce the size of the lesion. It should be remembered that many patients find dressing change a major ordeal which leaves them feeling very tired.

Odour is probably the problem that causes the greatest distress to patients. It is mostly due to bacterial invasion, although exuding necrotic wounds may also be offensive. A wound swab will identify the invading bacteria, so that appropriate systemic antibiotics can be prescribed. Topical agents can also be used. Hampson (1996) reviewed the use of metronidazole for malodorous wounds. To date the studies have been poor with inadequate numbers. However, it is widely used to reduce odour. Silver sulphadiazine cream can be used for *Pseudomonas aeruginosa* infections.

If the odour cannot be reduced, or even while action is being taken to reduce odour, other steps can be taken. The aim is to mask the smell. This can be achieved in a variety of ways. Activated charcoal dressings can be effective in absorbing odour (Lawrence *et al.*, 1993). They are often used in conjunction with other dressings. Air fresheners can help and stoma therapists can give advice on the use of deodorant solutions used by ostomists.

Copious exudate is another problem that concerns patients. Very absorbent dressings are necessary to provide comfort and dryness for the patient. Alginates and hydrocellular foams can be effective in controlling exudate. Grocott (1997, 1998) has undertaken a longitudinal multiple case design study to monitor the outcomes when using different dressings to manage exudate. She considers that the factor of greatest importance is fitting conformable dressing materials to the wound, thus reducing the risk of leakage. Dressing bulk can be reduced by the use of outer dressings with high moisture vapour transfer rates.

When aggressive treatment is suitable, wound debridement is a treatment option. Removal of necrotic or sloughy tissue can reduce odour and exudate. The quickest method is surgical debridement. This must be done by a skilled surgeon because of the distorted anatomy and the risk of capillary bleeding. Surgical debridement is not a suitable option for patients with a history of capillary bleeding into the wound. A variety of wound management products can be used, depending on the amount of exudate. Alginates and beads can be used on heavily exuding wounds. When there is moderate to low exudate, an amorphous hydrogel and occasionally hydrocolloids can be used. The position, size and spread of the lesion can affect dressing choice.

Capillary bleeding can be frightening for both the patient and the nurse. When there is a history of capillary bleeding, great care should be taken when removing the old dressing. If the dressing is adherent, it should be soaked with saline before removal is attempted. It may also be necessary to remove the dressing slowly in stages. It is better to take a long time to remove a dressing than to start bleeding which is difficult to control.

To control profuse bleeding, adrenaline can be applied directly to the wound. However, it should be used with caution, under medical supervision. Alginate dressings are useful when there is oozing. They can be removed easily by washing away with saline. If there is persistent bleeding, the haemoglobin should be checked regularly. Blood transfusions may be necessary to treat anaemia.

If radiotherapy treatment is being given to the lesion, attention must be paid to dressing selection. A range of dressings have been found to be suitable, including charcoal dressings, alginates and an amorphous hydrogel.

Dressing retention may be a problem. Ideally, the dressing should not be too bulky because it makes the wearing of clothes difficult and the patient becomes very self-conscious. Bandages and tubular net and tubular gauze are probably the most versatile means of dressing retention. Tape should be used with care as the skin may become sore with repeated dressing change. If the patient is undergoing a course of radiotherapy to the lesion, it may be necessary for the outer dressing to be removed for treatment. Again, the skin may become sore. 'Garments' made from tubular net allow easy access to the wound and will not further damage the skin.

Patients with lymphoedema may have been told that nothing can be done to reduce the swelling. This is not true. Although it is not possible to cure lymph-oedema, it can be controlled. Management of lymphoedema involves a four-fold plan and considerable commitment from the patient and, possibly, a member of the family. It is possible to reduce a severely swollen limb to a reasonable size and so improve the quality of life of the patient (Badger, 1987). Regnard et al. (1997) describe the cornerstones of treating lymphoedema as skin care, exercise and movement, truncal massage and support bandaging or hosiery.

Skin care is a vital aspect of overall care. Williams and Venables (1996) describe the need for daily washing and careful drying, especially between the digits. Creams should be applied to prevent the skin drying out and cracking. Over time, untreated lymphoedema will result in deep skin folds and ultimately hyperkeratosis. Emollients can help to prevent this occurring. Care should be taken to prevent the swollen limb getting burnt by the sun. Cuts and scratches can be a source of infection. They should be treated with antiseptic cream. Gloves should be worn for protection when working in the kitchen or garden. Jeffs (1993) has reviewed the effects of infection in lymphoedema. She suggests that *Streptococcus* is generally the causative organism. The infection should be treated with appropriate antibiotics.

Exercise assists in improving drainage of lymph from the limb. Muscle movement alters tissue pressure and has a massaging effect on the lymph vessels. The best effect is obtained if the exercises are carried out when the patient is wearing compression bandages or hosiery. Exercise also prevents or reduces stiffness of the joints. Passive movements should be carried out if the limb is paralysed. All patients should be encouraged to move as much as possible, but lifting and carrying heavy weights should be avoided.

Massage encourages the flow of lymph away from the limb. Occasionally, the swelling may have spread beyond the limb into the trunk. Massage should start on the trunk, which should be free of lymphoedema, before moving to a lymphoe-dematous limb (Regnard et al., 1997); this creates a space for the lymph in the swollen limb to flow into. The massage then continues down the affected limb. The massage technique should be gentle, so that it does not stimulate blood flow into the limb and increase congestion. It may need to be a little firmer when tissue fibrosis is present. Ko et al. (1998) monitored the effects of treatment for 299 patients over a 12-month period. They found a 59.1% reduction in size in arms and 67.7% reduction in size in legs after initial treatment averaging 15.7 days. This was maintained in 88% of compliant patients. The noncompliant patients regained 33% of the initial reduction.

Compression can be provided by bandages or compression hosiery, such as a sleeve. In the initial stages of treatment, bandages assist in reducing limb size. In severe cases the digits as well as the hand and arm, or foot and leg, should be bandaged. Once the limb has been reduced to a reasonable size, compression hosiery can be used to maintain limb reduction.

Intermittent pneumatic compression may be helpful for some patients. It is used in addition to massage and not as an alternative. The type of compression that is most effective is the multichamber sequential pump. The best effect is obtained by clearing fluid from the trunk before commencing treatment.

It is important to provide encouragement to the patient to persevere with all aspects of this plan. None of these treatments is effective in isolation. Significant reduction of a swollen limb can only be achieved when all aspects of the treatment plan are implemented. Carroll and Rose (1992) demonstrated that this type of treatment regime reduced pain in the limb as well as limb volume. Williams *et al.* (1996) described the benefits of a lymphoedema service accessible to all.

● *Evaluation* ●

Evaluation of the management of fungating wounds should always consider whether the predetermined goals have been attained. Good documentation can be used to maintain a record of effective care, thus providing guidelines for the management of other patients. Managing a fungating wound and providing care for the patient require considerable nursing skills. More research is needed in order to be able to identify the most effective care.

REFERENCES

Allen, S. (1983) Hang the patient upside down from the ceiling – it works every time. *General Practitioner*, June 24, 40–41.

Anthony. D. (1996) Receiver operating characteristic analysis. *Nurse Researcher*, **4** (2), 75–88.

Badger, C. (1987) Lymphoedema: management of patients with advanced cancer. *Professional Nurse*, **2** (4), 100–102.

Baker, S.R., Stacey, M.C. (1994) Epidemiology of chronic leg ulcers in Australia. *Australia & New Zealand Journal of Surgery*, **64** (4), 258–261.

Bale, S., Banks, V., Haglestein, S., Harding, K.G. (1998) A comparison of two amorphous hydrogels in the debridement of pressure sores. *Journal of Wound Care*, **7** (2), 65–68.

Bale, S., Crook, H. (1998) The preliminary results of a comparative study on the performance characteristics of a new hydrogel versus an existing hydrogel on necrotic pressure ulcers, in (eds) Leaper, D., Cherry, G., Cockbill, S., Dealey, C., Flanagan, M., Hofman, D. *et al.*, *Proceedings of the EWMA/Journal of Wound Care Spring Meeting*. Macmillan Magazines Ltd, London.

Bale, S., Squires, D., Vernon, T., Walker, A., Benbow, M., Harding, K.G. (1997) A comparison of two dressings in pressure sore management. *Journal of Wound Care*, **6** (10), 463–466.

Barczak, C.A., Barnett, R.I., Childs, E.J., Bosley, L.M. (1997) Fourth national pressure ulcer prevalence survey. *Advanced Wound Care*, **10** (4), 18–26.

Barrois, B., Allaert, F.A., Colin, D. (1998) Epidemiology and pressure sores, in (eds) Leaper, D., Cherry, G., Cockbill, S., Dealey, C., Flanagan, M., Hofman, D., *et al.*, *Proceedings of the EWMA/Journal of Wound Care Spring Meeting*. Macmillan Magazines Ltd, London.

Bergstrom, N., Braden, B., Brandt, J., Krall, K. (1985) Adequacy of descriptive scales for reporting diet intake in the institutionalised elderly. *Journal of Nutrition for the Elderly*, **6** (1), 3–16.

Bergstrom, N., Braden, B., Laguzza, A. (1987) The Braden scale for predicting pressure sore risk. *Nursing Research*, **36** (4), 205–210.

Berlowitz, D.R., Wilking, S.V.B. (1989) Risk factors for pressure sores: a comparison of cross-sectional and cohort-derived data. *Journal of the American Geriatric Society*, **37**, 1043–1050.

Blair, S.D., Wright, D.D.I., Backhouse, C.M., Riddle, E., McCollum, C.N. (1988) Sustained compression and healing of chronic leg ulcers. *British Medical Journal*, **297** (6657), 1159–1161.

Bliss, M. (1990) Editorial – Preventing pressure sores. *Lancet*, **335**, 1311–1312.

Bliss, M., Schofield, M. (1993) A pilot leg ulcer clinic in a geriatric day hospital. *Age and Aging*, **22**, 279–284.

Bliss, M.R., Thomas, J.M. (1993) Clinical trials with budgetry implications: establishing randomised trials of pressure relieving aids. *Professional Nurse*, **8** (5), 292–296.

Bosanquet, N. (1992) Costs of venous ulcers: from maintenance therapy to investment programmes. *Phlebology*, **7**, suppl. 1, 44–46.

Brandeis, G.H., Ooi, W.L., Hossain, M., Morris, J.N., Lipsitz, L.A. (1994) A longitudinal study of risk factors associated with the formation of pressure ulcers in nursing homes. *Journal of the American Geriatric Society*, **42**, 388–393.

Bridel, J. (1993a) Assessing the risk of pressure sores. *Nursing Standard*, **7** (25), 32–35.

Bridel, J. (1993b) Pressure sore risk in operating theatres. *Nursing Standard*, **7** (32 Suppl.), 4–10.

Brooks, R., Thomson, J. (1997) Pressure area care and estimating the cost of pressure sores: Critique 2. *Journal of Wound Care*, **6** (3), 135–137.

Buss, I.C., Halfens, R.J., Abu-Saad, H.H. (1997) The effectiveness of massage in preventing pressure sores: a literature review. *Rehabilitation Nursing*, **22** (5), 229–234.

Callam, M.J., Ruckley, C.V., Harper, D.R., Dale, J.J. (1985) Chronic ulceration of the leg: extent of the problems and provision of care. *British Medical Journal*, **290**, 1855–1856.

Cameron, J. (1998) Skin care for patients with chronic leg ulcers. *Journal of Wound Care*, **7** (9), 459–462.

Carroll, D., Rose, K. (1992) Treatment leads to significant improvement: effects of conservative treatment on pain in lymphoedema. *Professional Nurse*, **8** (1), 32–36.

Chase, S.K., Melloni, M., Savage, A. (1997) A forever healing: the lived experience of venous ulcer disease. *Journal of Vascular Nursing*, **15** (2), 73–78.

Clark, M., Cullum, N. (1992) Matching patient need for pressure sore prevention with the supply of pressure redistributing mattresses. *Journal of Advanced Nursing*, **17**, 310–316.

Clough, N.P. (1994) The cost of pressure area management in an intensive care unit. *Journal of Wound Care*, **3** (1), 33–35.

Colin, D., Dizien, O., Yvon, C. (1997) The clinical investigation of a transparent semipermeable adhesive film dressing with an extra-thin hydrocolloid in the management of stage I and II pressure sores, in (eds) Leaper, D.J., Cherry, G.W., Dealey, C., Lawrence, J.C., Turner, T.D., *Proceedings of the 6th European Conference on Advances in Wound Management*. Macmillan Magazines Ltd, London.

Colin, D., Kurring, P.A., Quinlan, D., Yvon, C. (1996) The clinical investigation of an amorphous hydrogel compared with a dextranomer paste dressing in the management of sloughy pressure sores, in (eds) Cherry, G.W., Gottrup, F., Lawrence, J.C., Moffatt, C.J., Turner, T.D., *Proceedings of the 5th European Conference on Advances in Wound Management*. Macmillan Magazines Ltd, London.

Conference Report (1990) Diabetes mellitus in Europe: a problem at all ages and in all countries. A model for prevention and self care. *Diabetic Medicine*, **70**, 360.

Connor, H. (1997) The St Vincent amputation target: the cost of achieving it and the cost of failure. *Practical Diabetes International*, **14** (6), 152–153.

Cornwall, J.V., Dore, C.J., Lewis, J.D. (1986) Leg ulcers: epidemiology and aetiology. *British Medical Journal*, **73**, 693–696.

Culley, F. (1998) Nursing aspects of pressure sore prevention and therapy. *British Journal of Nursing*, **7** (15), 879–884.

Cullum, N., Clark, M. (1992) Intrinsic factors associated with pressure sores in elderly people. *Journal of Advanced Nursing*, **17**, 427–431.

Dale, J., Gibson, B. (1986) Leg ulcers: a disease affecting all ages. *Professional Nurse*, **1** (8), 213–217.

Dale, J., Gibson, B. (1990) Back-up for the venous pump. *Professional Nurse*, **5** (9), 481–486.

Danchaivijitr, S., Suthisanon, L., Jitreecheue, L., Tantiwatanapaibool, Y. (1995) *Journal of the Medical Association of Thailand*, **78**, suppl. 1, S1–S6.

David, J.A., Chapman, R.G., Chapman, E.J., Lockett, B. (1983) *An Investigation of the Current Methods used in Nursing for the Care of Patients with Established Pressure Sores*. Nursing Practice Research Unit, Northwick Park, Middlesex.

Dealey, C. (1991a) The size of the pressure sore problem in a teaching hospital. *Journal of Advanced Nursing*, **16**, 663–670.

Dealey, C. (1991b) Causes of leg ulcers. *Nursing*, **4** (35), 23–24.

Dealey, C. (1993) Pressure sores; the result of bad nursing? *British Journal of Nursing*, **1** (15), 748.

Dealey, C. (1997) *Managing Pressure Sore Prevention*. Mark Allen Publishing Ltd, Salisbury.

Dealey, C., Earwaker, T., Eden, L. (1991) Are your patients sitting comfortably? *Journal of Tissue Viability*, **1** (2), 36–39.

Dealey, C., Keogh, A. (1998) A randomised study comparing the Triple Care cleanser and cream system with soap and water for elderly incontinent patients, in (eds) Leaper, D., Dealey, C., Franks, P.J., Hofman, D., Moffatt, C.J., *Proceedings of the 7th European Conference on Advances in Wound Management*. EMAP Healthcare Ltd, London.

Deeks, J.J. (1996) Pressure sore prevention: using and evaluating risk assessment tools. *British Journal of Nursing*, **5** (5), 313–320.

Department of Health (1992) *Health of the Nation*. HMSO, London.

Department of Health (1993) *Pressure Sores: A Key Quality Indicator*. Department of Health, London.

Dyson, R. (1978) Bed sores – the injuries hospital staff inflict on patients. *Nursing Mirror*, **146**, 30–32.

Ebbeskog, R., Lindholm, C., Ohman, S. (1996) Leg and foot ulcer patients. Epidemiology and nursing care in an urban population in south Stockholm, Sweden. *Scandinavian Journal of Primary Health Care*, **14** (4), 238–243.

Effective Health Care (1995) The prevention and treatment of pressure sores. *Effective Health Care Bulletin*, **2** (1), 1–16.

Ek, A.C., Gustavssen, G., Lewis, D.H. (1987) Skin blood flow in relation to external pressure and temperature in the supine position on a standard hospital mattress. *Scandinavian Journal of Rehabilitation*, **19**, 121–126.

European Pressure Ulcer Advisory Panel (1998) A policy statement on the prevention of pressure ulcers from the European Pressure Ulcer Advisory Panel. *British Journal of Nursing*, **7** (15), 888–890.

Exton-Smith, A.N., Sherwin, R.W. (1961) The prevention of pressure sores: the significance of spontaneous bodily movement. *Lancet*, **II**, 1124–1126.

Fentem, P.H. (1986) Elastic hosiery. *Pharmacy Update*, **5**, 200–205.

Flanagan, M. (1997) Choosing pressure sore risk assessment tools. *Professional Nurse*, **12** (6 Suppl.), 3–7.

Fletcher, A., Cullum, N., Sheldon, T. (1997) A systematic review of compression treatment for venous leg ulcers. *British Medical Journal*, **315**, 576–580.

Foster, A. (1997) Psychological aspects of treating the diabetic foot. *Practical Diabetes International*, **14** (2), 56–58.

Fowler, E. (1990) Chronic wounds: an overview, in (ed) Krasner, D., *Chronic Wound Care: a Clinical Sourcebook for Healthcare Professionals*. Health Management Publications Inc., King of Prussia, Pennsylvania.

Franks, P.J., Oldroyd, M.I., Dickson, D., Sharp, E.J., Moffatt, C.J. (1995) Risk factors for leg ulcer recurrence: a randomised trial of two types of compression stocking. *Age and Aging*, **24**, 490–494.

Gebhardt, K. (1995) What causes pressure sores? *Nursing Standard*, **9** (suppl. 31), 48–51.

General, Municipal and Boilermakers Union (1985) *Hazard in the Health Service – An A–Z Guide*. GMB, London.

Gilchrist, B. (1989) Treating leg ulcers. *Nursing Times Community Outlook*, **85** (6 Suppl.), 25–26.

Grey, J.E., Lowe, G., Bale, S., Harding K.G. (1998) The use of cultured dermis in the treatment of diabetic foot ulcers. *Journal of Wound Care*, **7** (7), 324–325.

Grocott, P. (1995) The palliative management of fungating malignant wounds. *Journal of Wound Care*, **4** (5), 240–242.

Grocott, P. (1997) Evaluation of a tool to assess the management of fungating wounds. *Journal of Wound Care*, **6** (9), 421–424.

Grocott, P. (1998) Exudate management in fungating wounds. *Journal of Wound Care*, **7** (9), 445–448.

Gruen, R.L., Chang, S., MacLellan, D.G. (1996) Optimising the hospital management of leg ulcers. *Australia & New Zealand Journal of Surgery*, **66** (3), 171–174.

Hampson, J.P. (1996) The use of metronidazole in the treatment of malodorous wounds. *Journal of Wound Care*, **5** (9), 421–425.

Harkiss, K.J. (1985) Cost analysis of dressing materials used in venous leg ulcers. *Pharmaceutical Journal*, **235** (6344), 268–269.

Hawkins, J.E. (1997) The effectiveness of pressure-reducing table pads as an intervention to reduce the risk of intraoperatively acquired pressure sores. *Military Medicine*, **162** (11), 759–761.

Health and Safety Executive (1992) *Manual Handling: Manual Handling Operations Regulations. Guidance on Regulations*. HSE, London.

Hibbs, P. (1988) *Pressure Area Care for the City and Hackney Health Authority*. City and Hackney Health Authority, London.

Hitch, S. (1995) NHS Executive Nursing Directorate – strategy for major clinical guidelines – prevention and management of pressure sores, a literature review. *Journal of Tissue Viability*, **5** (1), 3–24.

Hofman, D., Ryan, T.J., Arnold, F., Cherry, G.W., Lindholm, C., Bjellerup, M., Glynn, C. (1997) Pain in venous leg ulcers. *Journal of Wound Care*, **6** (5), 222–224.

Ivetic, O., Lyne, P.A. (1990) Fungating and ulcerating malignant lesions: a review of the literature. *Journal of Advanced Nursing*, **15**, 83–88.

Jay, R. (1997) Other considerations in selecting a support surface. *Advanced Wound Care*, **10** (7), 37–42.

Jeffs, E. (1993) The effect of acute inflammatory episodes on the treatment of lymphoedema. *Journal of Tissue Viability*, **3** (2), 51–55.

Jones, J.E., Nelson, E.A. (1998) Compression hosiery in the management of venous leg ulcers. *Journal of Wound Care*, **7** (6), 293–296.

Jordan, M.M., Clark, M. (1977) *Report on Incidence of Pressure Sores in the Patient*

Community of the Greater Glasgow Health Board Area. University of Strathclyde, Jan. 21.

Kabagambe, M.K., Swain, I., Shakespeare, P. (1994) An investigation of the effects on the microcirculation of the skin (reactive hyperaemia) in spinal cord injured patients. *Journal of Tissue Viability*, **4** (4), 110–123.

Khoo, C., Bailey, B.N. (1990) Reconstructive surgery, in (ed) Bader, D., *Pressure Sores – Clinical Practice and Scientific Approach.* Macmillan Press, London.

Kierney, P.C., Engrav, L.H., Isik, F.F., Esselman, P.C., Cardenas, D.D., Rand, R.P. (1998) Results of 268 pressure sores in 158 patients managed jointly by plastic surgery and rehabilitation medicine. *Plastic and Reconstructive Surgery*, **102** (3), 765–772.

Ko, D.S., Lerner, K., Klose, G., Cosimi, A.B. (1998) Effective treatment of lymphoedema of the extremities. *Archives of Surgery*, **133** (4), 452–458.

Krouskop, M. (1983) A synthesis of the factors which contribute to pressure sore formation. *Medical Hypothesis*, **11**, 255–267.

Landis, E.M. (1931) Micro-injection studies of capillary blood pressure in human skin. *Heart*, **15**, 209–228.

Lapsley, H.M., Vogels, R. (1996) Cost and prevention of pressure ulcer in an acute teaching hospital. *International Journal for Quality in Health Care*, **8** (1), 61–66.

Lawrence, J.C., Lilly, H.A., Kidson, A. (1993) Malodour and dressings containing active charcoal, in (eds) Harding, K.G., Cherry, G., Dealey, C., Turner, T.D., *Proceedings of the 2nd European Conference on Advances in Wound Management.* Macmillan Magazines Ltd, London.

Litchfield, B., Ramkissoon, S. (1996) Foot-care education in patients with diabetes. *Professional Nurse*, **11** (8), 510–512.

Lockett, B. (1983) Prevalence and incidence in pressure sore disease, *Symposium at Royal Hospital and Home for Incurables.*

Logan, R.A., Thomas, S., Harding, E.F., Collyer, G.J. (1992) A comparison of sub-bandage pressures produced by experienced and inexperienced bandagers. *Journal of Wound Care*, **1** (3), 23–26.

Logan, V. (1995) Incidence and prevalence of lymphoedema: a literature review. *Journal of Clinical Nursing*, **4** (4), 213–219.

Loudon, I.S.L. (1982) Leg ulcers in the eighteenth and early nineteenth centuries. *Journal of the Royal College of General Practitioners*, **32**, 301–309.

Lowthian, P. (1979) Turning clocks, a system to prevent pressure sores. *Nursing Mirror*, **148** (21), 30–31.

Magazinovic, N., Phillips-Turner, J., Wilson, G.V. (1993) Assessing nurses' knowledge of bandages and bandaging. *Journal of Wound Care*, **2** (2), 97–101.

Masson, E.A., Angle, S., Roseman, P., Soper, C., Wilson, I., Cotton, M., Boulton, A.J.M. (1989) Diabetic ulcers – do patients know how to protect themselves? *Practical Diabetes*, **6** (1), 22–23.

Mayberry, J.C., Moneta, G.L., Taylor, L.M., Porter, J.M. (1991) Fifteen-year results of ambulatory compression therapy for chronic venous ulcers. *Surgery*, **109** (5), 575–581.

Mulder, G., Robison, J., Seeley, J. (1990) Study of sequential compression therapy in the treatment of non-healing chronic venous ulcers. *Wounds*, **2** (3), 111–115.

National Pressure Ulcer Advisory Panel (1989) Pressure ulcers prevalence, cost and risk assessment. *Decubitus*, **2** (2), 24–28.

Nelzen, O., Bergqvist, D., Lindhagen, A., Hallbook, T. (1991) Chronic leg ulcers: an underestimated problem in primary health care among elderly patients. *Journal of Epidemiology and Community Health*, **45** (3), 184–187.

Nightingale, F. (1861) *Notes on Nursing.* Appleton Century, New York.

Norton, D., Mclaren, R., Exton-Smith, A.N. (1975) *An Investigation of Geriatric Nursing Problems.* Churchill Livingstone, Edinburgh.

Nyquist, R., Hawthorn, P.J. (1987) The prevalence of pressure sores in an area health authority. *Journal of Advanced Nursing,* **12**, 183–187.

Nyquist, R., Hawthorn, P.J. (1988) The incidence of pressure sores amongst a group of elderly patients with fractured neck of femur. *Care – Science and Practice,* **6** (1), 3–7.

O'Brien, S.P., Wind, S., van Rijswijk, L., Kerstein, M.D. (1998) Sequential biannual prevalence studies of pressure ulcers at Allegheny-Hahnemann University Hospital. *Ostomy and Wound Management,* **44** (3A Suppl.), 78S-88S.

O'Dea, K. (1993) Prevalence of pressure damage in hospital patients in the UK. *Journal of Wound Care,* **2** (4), 221–225.

O'Dea, K. (1995) Prevalence of pressure sores in four European countries. *Journal of Wound Care,* **4** (4), 192–195.

Oertwich, P.A., Kindshuh, A.M., Bergstrom, N. (1995) The effects of small shifts in body weight on blood flow and interface pressure. *Research in Nursing & Health,* **18**, 481–488.

Pinchkofsky-Devin, G., Kaminski, M.V. (1986) Correlation of pressure sores and nutritional status. *Journal of the American Geriatric Society,* **34**, 435–440.

Podmore, J. (1993) Report on Tissue Viability Society Spring Conference. *Nursing Standard,* **7** (32 Suppl.), 14.

Preston, K.W. (1988) Positioning for comfort and pressure relief: the 30 degree alternative. *Care – Science and Practice,* **6** (4), 116–119.

Ray, S.A., Minty, I., Buckenham, T.M. (1995) Clinical outcome and restenosis following PTA for ischaemic rest pain or ulceration.

Regan, M.B., Byers, P.H., Mayrovitz, H.N. (1995) Efficacy of a comprehensive pressure ulcer prevention programme in an extended care facility. *Advances in Wound Care,* **8** (3), 49–55.

Regnard, C., Allport, S., Stephenson, L. (1997) ABC of palliative care: mouthcare, skin care and lymphoedema. *British Medical Journal,* **315**, 1002–1005.

Rithalia, S.V.S. (1989) Comparison of pressure distribution in wheelchair seat cushions. *Care – Science and Practice,* **7** (4), 87–89.

Rosen, T. (1980) Cutaneous metastases. *Medical Clinics of North America,* **64** (5), 885–900.

Royal College of Nursing (1996) *RCN Code of Practice for Patient Handling.* Royal College of Nursing, London.

Ryan, T.J. (1987) *The Management of Leg Ulcers,* 2nd edn. Oxford University Press, Oxford.

Sanada, H., Nagakawa, T., Yamamoto, M., Higashidani, K., Tsuru, H., Sugama, J. (1997) The role of blood flow in pressure ulcer development during surgery. *Advances in Wound Care,* **10** (6), 29–34.

Sandeman, D.D., Pym, C.A., Green, E.M., Seamark, C., Shoare, A.C., Tooke, J.E. (1991) Microvascular vasodilation in the feet of newly diagnosed non-insulin dependent diabetics. *British Medical Journal,* **302** (6785), 1122–1123.

Schnelle, J.F., Adamson, J.M., Cruise, P.A., Al-Samarrai, N., Sarbaugh, F.C., Uman, G., Ouslander, J.G. (1997) Skin disorders and moisture in incontinent nursing home residents: intervention implications. *Journal of the American Geriatric Society,* **45**, 1182–1188.

Schraibman, I.G. (1987) The bacteriology of leg ulcers. *Phlebology,* **2** (4), 265–269.

Scottish Intercollegiate Guidelines Network (1997) *Management of Diabetic Foot Disease.* Scottish Intercollegiate Guidelines Network, Edinburgh.

Seeley, J., Jensen, J.L., Vigil, S. (1998) A 40-patient randomised clinical trial to compare the performance of Allevyn Adhesive hydrocellular dressing and a hydrocolloid in the management of pressure ulcers, in (eds) Leaper, D., Dealey, C., Franks, P.J., Hofman, D., Moffatt, C.J., *Proceedings of the 7th European Conference on Advances in Wound Management.* EMAP Healthcare Ltd, London.

Simon, D.A., Freak, L., Kinsella, A., Walsh, J., Lane, C., Groarke, L., McCollum, C. (1996) Community leg ulcer clinics: a comparative study in two health authorities. *British Medical Journal,* **312**, 1648–1651.

Sims, R., Fitzgerald, V. (1985) *Community Nursing Management of Patients with Ulcerating/fungating Breast Disease.* Royal College of Nursing, London.

Sopata, M. (1997) A comparative, prospective study of the treatment of stage II and III pressure sores in patients with advanced cancer: Aquagel versus Lyofoam A., in (eds) Leaper, D.J., Cherry, G.W., Dealey, C., Lawrence, J.C., Turner, T.D., *Proceedings of the 6th European Conference on Advances in Wound Management.* Macmillan Magazines Ltd, London.

Stemmer, R. (1969) Ambulatory elasto-compressive treatment of the lower extremities particularly with elastic stockings. *Der Kassenatzt,* **9**, 1–8.

Stordeur, S., Laurent, S., D'Hoore, W. (1998) The importance of repeated risk assessment for pressure sores in cardiovascular surgery. *Journal of Cardiovascular Surgery (Torino),* **39** (3), 343–349.

Teot, L., N'Guyen, C., Leglise, S., Gavroy, J.P., Handshuh, R. (1998a) Safety and efficacy of a new hydrocolloid in the treatment of stage I and II pressure sores, in (eds) Leaper, D., Cherry, G., Cockbill, S., Dealey, C., Flanagan, M., Hofman, D., *et al.*, *Proceedings of the EWMA/Journal of Wound Care Spring Meeting.* Macmillan Magazines Ltd, London.

Teot, L., Richard, D., Votte, A., Dare, F., Eyssette, M., Strubel, D., *et al.* (1998b) Comparison of an Aquacel dressing regime and a traditional dressing regime in the management of pressure sores, in (eds) Leaper, D., Cherry, G., Cockbill, S., Dealey, C., Flanagan, M., Hofman, D., *et al. Proceedings of the EWMA/Journal of Wound Care Spring Meeting.* Macmillan Magazines Ltd, London.

Thomas, S. (1990) Bandages and bandaging. *Nursing Standard,* **4** (39 Suppl.), 4–6.

Thomas, S. (1992) *Current Practices in the Management of Fungating Lesions and Radiation Damaged Skin.* Surgical Materials Testing Laboratory, Bridgend.

Thomas, S., Banks, V., Bale, S., Fear-Price, M., Hagelstein, S., Harding, K.G., *et al.* (1997) A comparison of two dressings in the management of chronic wounds. *Journal of Wound Care,* **6** (8), 383–386.

Tingle, J. (1997) Pressure sores: counting the legal cost of nursing neglect. *British Journal of Nursing,* **6** (13), 757–758.

Touche Ross & Co. (1993) *The Costs of Pressure Sores.* Department of Health, London.

Versluysen, M. (1986) How elderly patients with femoral fractures develop pressure sores in hospital. *British Medical Journal,* **292**, 1311–1313.

Wagner, F.W. (1981) The dysvascular foot: a system for diagnosis and treatment. *Foot Ankle,* **2**, 64.

Walters, D.P., Gatling, W., Hill, R.D., Mullee, M.A. (1993) The prevalence of foot deformity in diabetic subjects: a population study in an English community. *Practical Diabetes,* **10** (3), 106–108.

Waterlow, J. (1985) A risk assessment card. *Nursing Times,* **81** (48), 49–55.

Waterlow, J. (1988) Prevention is cheaper than cure. *Nursing Times,* **84** (25), 69–70.

Werngren-Elgstrom, M., Lidman, D. (1994) Lymphoedema of the lower extremities after surgery and radiotherapy for cancer of the cervix. *Scandinavian Journal of Plastic & Reconstructive Surgery & Hand Surgery*, **28** (4), 289–293.

Williams, A., Venables, J. (1996) Skin care in patients with uncomplicated lymphoedema. *Journal of Wound Care*, **5** (5), 223–226.

Williams, A.E., Bergl, S., Twycross, R.G. (1996) A 5-year review of a lymphoedema service. *European Journal of Cancer Care (Engl)*, **5** (1), 56–59.

Young, J. (1992) The use of specialised beds and mattresses. *Journal of Tissue Viability*, **2** (3), 79–81.

Young, M.J., Boulton, A.J.M. (1991) Guidelines for identifying the at-risk foot. *Practical Diabetes*, **8** (3), 103–105.

Young, T., Williams, C., Benbow, M., Collier, M., Banks, V., Jones, H. (1997) A study of two hydrogels used in the management of pressure sores, in (eds) Leaper, D.J., Cherry, G.W., Dealey, C., Lawrence, J.C., Turner, T.D., *Proceedings of the 6th European Conference on Advances in Wound Management*. Macmillan Magazines Ltd, London.

Zernikern, W. (1994) Preventing heel pressure sores: a comparison of heel pressure relieving devices. *Journal of Clinical Nursing*, **3**, 375–380.

Chapter 6
The Management of Patients with Acute Wounds

6.1 INTRODUCTION

Acute wounds can be defined as wounds of sudden onset and of short duration. They include surgical wounds and traumatic wounds such as burns. Acute wounds can occur in people of all ages and generally heal easily without complication. This section will consider the specific care needed for patients with acute wounds.

6.2 THE CARE OF SURGICAL WOUNDS

Surgical wounds are, by their very nature, premeditated wounds. This allows the surgeon to attempt to reduce any risks of complication to a minimum. However, as increasingly sophisticated surgery is performed, often on relatively elderly patients, complications are still a hazard. One aspect of nursing care is to monitor the progress of the wound, so that there is an early identification of any problems.

6.2.1 The management of surgical wounds

● *Patient assessment* ●

This is essential to identify any factors that can affect healing. This topic is covered in more detail in Chapter 2. Potential problem areas include:

Maintaining a safe environment   the risk of infection must be considered.
Communicating   identify patient understanding of the operative procedure. Postoperative pain must be assessed and controlled.
Breathing   recording of vital signs for indication of haemorrhage.
Eating and drinking   assessment of nutritional status is essential as patients may be starved for long periods.
Controlling body temperature   pyrexia is an indication of infection.
Mobilising   mobility is often reduced in the postoperative period.
Expressing sexuality   assess patients' reaction to their altered body image.
Sleeping   sleeping patterns may be altered because of pain and/or disturbance by nursing staff.
Psychological care   particular problems which may be identified are fear and powerlessness.

Spiritual care   spiritual distress may be caused by loss of meaning or purpose in life.

● *Wound assessment* ●

This should identify the method of closure, note the use of any drains and observe for any indication of complication. Westaby (1985) describes the main aim of surgical wound closure as being the restoration of function and physical integrity with the minimum deformity and without infection. The method of wound closure is selected in order to achieve this aim and it will vary according to the surgery performed. There are three methods of closure: primary closure, delayed primary closure and healing by second intention.

Primary closure

Hippocrates (460–377 BC) was the first to describe this method of wound closure. He called it healing by first intention. The skin edges are held in approximation by sutures, clips, staples or tape. In these wounds the skin edges seal very quickly, first with fibrin from clot formation and then as epithelialisation occurs. Within 48 hours the wound should be totally sealed, thus preventing the ingress of bacteria.

● *Nursing care* ●

The care of wounds healing by first intention is generally straightforward. A simple island dressing is commonly used to cover the wound at the end of the operation. Several studies have shown that the dressing can be removed after 24–48 hours and need not be replaced (Cruse & Foord, 1980; Weiss, 1983; Chrintz et al., 1989). Some surgeons prefer to cover the wound with a film dressing and leave it in place until the sutures are removed. Whichever method is used, normal hygiene can be resumed and the patient may bath or shower.

Uncomplicated healing may not be the only factor to consider in wound management. Briggs (1996) undertook a small study where 30 patients were randomised to either a dry dressing removed after 48 hours or a film dressing left in place until suture removal. She found a significant difference in pain on day three after the dry dressing had been removed. Those with no dressing had sufficient pain to require analgesia. Holm et al. (1997) randomly allocated 73 patients to either a thin hydrocolloid dressing or a dry dressing removed after 48 hours. They found no difference between the two groups in respect of healing or the cosmetic appearance of the scar. However, the hydrocolloid group appeared to mobilise and return to normal daily activities more quickly. One conclusion might be that patients in the hydrocolloid group had less pain and so were able to move more freely. This concept is worthy of further study.

The wound should be monitored daily for any indication of complication. Removal of sutures or other types of wound closure is usually carried out under medical supervision.

Delayed primary closure

This method of closure is used when there has been considerable bacterial contamination. Initially, any body cavity is closed and the remaining tissue layers are left open to allow free drainage of pus. After about five days, these layers are closed and the wound will heal as any primarily closed wound. Wound drains may be used to assist in the removal of any fluid remaining at the wound base.

● *Nursing Care* ●

The aim of management of these wounds is to allow free drainage of any pus. This may be achieved by loose packing of the cavity. As the wound will be sutured at about day five, the promotion of granulation is not a major aim. If ribbon gauze is used, it should be kept moist and changed regularly to prevent it drying out and adhering to the wound. Alginate rope may also be used as it is very absorbent and can be removed without pain to the patient. Once the wound is sutured it should be treated as a wound healing by first intention.

Healing by second intention

Healing by second intention describes a wound that is left open and heals by granulation, contraction and epithelialisation. This method may be used for a variety of reasons:

(a)   There may be considerable tissue loss, e.g. radical vulvectomy.
(b)   The surgical incision is shallow, but has a large surface area, e.g. donor sites.
(c)   There may have been infection (for example a ruptured appendix) or an abscess may have been drained, and free drainage of any pus is essential.

● *Nursing care* ●

The care of various types of surgical wounds will be described here.

Surgical cavities

Surgical cavities are generally clean wounds with a healthy bed which would be expected to heal without complication. Harding (1990) suggests that surgical cavities should be boat-shaped in order to heal rapidly without premature surface healing. Simple wound measurement is usually sufficient to monitor healing rates (see Section 3.3). The wound should also be observed for indications of infection.

Selection of a suitable dressing depends on the position of the wound and the amount of exudate. Traditionally, ribbon gauze packing, often soaked in antiseptic solutions, has been used in these wounds. Ricci *et al.* (1998) compared iodine-soaked gauze with a foam stent in patients following pilonidal sinus excision. They found the foam stent to be more effective; healing time was faster (median 33.5 days compared with 73 days), and the patients with the foam stent were able to return to work after 12 days compared with 23 days. Far fewer dressings were required – 20 foam stents compared with 868 gauze packs. In addition, the foam stent group had pain-free dressing changes whereas the gauze group found the dressing change painful and bleeding occurred. This small study clearly demonstrates the problems found with gauze packing.

Foam stents have been used for some considerable time in a variety of surgical cavities such as pilonidal sinus excision (Wood & Hughes, 1975, Marks et al., 1985). Like other modern products the dressings have been modified and improved over time. Bale (1997) undertook a non-comparative study of the third generation foam stent (Cavi-Care®). Fifty patients with surgical cavities were assessed. There was 60% healing at 12 weeks and the dressing was found to be comfortable and easy to insert and remove. Berry et al. (1996) compared a preformed foam stent with an alginate rope for 20 patients with pilonidal sinus excision. They found no significant difference between the two groups, with both dressings performing well. The researchers concluded that both types of dressings were suitable for cavity wounds.

Alginate rope and ribbon have been used successfully in cavity wounds. It is especially useful when there is a heavy exudate in the early stages of healing. Gupta et al. (1991) have found alginate ribbon less painful to remove in comparison with traditional gauze packing. Williams et al. (1995) compared two alginate rope dressings in surgical cavities. They found no differences between the two groups when considering healing, pain and ease of use.

Foster and Moore (1997) compared a second generation hydrocolloid hydrofibre dressing with proflavine-soaked gauze in 40 patients with a variety of surgical cavities. There was a significant difference between the two groups with the ribbon gauze group suffering more pain and the hydrofibre group finding dressing removal and application much easier.

Skin grafts

Skin grafts are widely used in reconstructive surgery following trauma or burns. They may also be used to repair chronic wounds such as pressure sores or leg ulcers. Skin grafting is a technique which permits the transfer of a portion of skin from one part of the body to another. There are several ways of classifying skin grafts. They can be divided into:

- Autografts   a graft of the patient's own skin.
- Allografts   a graft taken from another individual.
- Xenografts   a graft taken from another species.

Grafts can be described according to their thickness. This depends on the amount of dermis that is included in the graft. A full-thickness graft includes the epidermis and all the dermis. A partial- or split-thickness graft includes the epidermis and some dermis. This type of graft can be cut to varying thickness depending on need. The graft can also be meshed in order to cover a larger surface area.

Other types of graft are flaps or pedicle grafts, pinch grafts and tissue cultures. Flaps may include other tissue besides skin and one part of the graft is still attached to the original site. This provides a blood supply to the graft until a new blood supply has been established. It is particularly useful in areas where the blood supply is poor and for areas of the face. An example is a gluteal rotation flap to cover the cavity of an ischial pressure sore.

Pinch grafts are small pieces of skin which have been obtained by pinching the area with forceps or lifting with a needle and slicing off with a knife. They have been used as a method of treating leg ulcers. Ryan (1987) suggests that they are only moderately successful though, as more than half have recurrence within three months. This is because the underlying cause of ulceration remains unchanged.

Tissue culture has been developed primarily in burns units, where repeated grafting from the same donor site may be necessary for patients with large surface area burns. A small sample of skin about 2 cm in diameter can be used to culture epithelial sheets many times this size. One of the early studies was carried out by Gallico *et al.* (1984) on two children who had burn injuries affecting more than 95% of their body surface area. Tissue culture provided effective grafts for more than 50% of the body surface. When such extensive burns occur, autografting is very limited because of the lack of appropriate donor sites. Allografts are also used, but they do not always take. Tissue culture can reduce the need for frequent surgery to take further grafts.

Grafts may be sutured or stapled in position or just laid in place. The graft may be left exposed or covered with a dressing to help anchor it in place. The graft must be observed carefully for any indication of infection, oedema or haematoma. It may also be necessary to immobilise the area so that the graft does not slip out of position. Tension over the graft must also be avoided as it may damage the vulnerable blood supply.

A gauze dressing is commonly used to cover the graft. If the dressing is removed, it must be done extremely carefully in order to avoid loosening the graft. Davey (1997a) described the use of Hyperfix® in a paediatric burns unit over a 12-year period. It was used for more than 500 grafts and found to be an effective covering. Peanut oil was routinely applied to the strapping two hours before dressing change in order to facilitate its removal without damage to the graft. Platt *et al.* (1996) undertook a small randomised trial comparing the use of a silicone net dressing with paraffin gauze. There was no difference in graft take between the two groups. However, the silicone net group had significantly less pain at dressing change and the dressing was easier to remove than the paraffin gauze.

As vascularisation of the graft occurs, it becomes approximately the same colour as the donor site. In Caucasians, the ideal colour is pink. It is more difficult to assess the vascularity of a graft in darker skins. Coull and Wylie (1990) suggest the use of a colour code along with an assessment chart to monitor the progress of skin flaps.

Once a graft has taken, it still needs to be handled very carefully as the tissues remain fragile. It should be protected against any extremes of temperature and sunlight. After the graft has healed the skin should be massaged twice daily with a bland moisturising cream. This helps to improve the suppleness of the skin as it is likely to be less well lubricated than normal. Plate 28 illustrates the discoloration and dryness of healed mesh graft sites.

A graft may fail to take for a variety of reasons. If there is an inadequate blood supply to the graft bed the microcirculation will fail to grow into the graft and it will necrose from lack of oxygen. Equally, haematoma formation will cause separation of the graft. If the graft slides out of position it will cause separation of some or all of the graft and lead to failure.

Infection, especially from *Pseudomonas aeruginosa* and β-haemolytic *Streptococcus*, will also cause failure. Infection will cause pain, odour, itching and redness around the edges of the graft and a low-grade fever (Francis, 1998). It is most likely to occur between the second and fourth postoperative day.

Donor sites

Ideally, donor sites are taken from a part of the body where the skin provides a good match for the recipient site. The colour, texture and hair-bearing properties of the skin have to be considered. One of the commonest areas for a donor site is the thigh, where a large area of skin can be obtained.

Donor sites are often described as being more painful than the skin graft for which the removed skin has been used. This is probably, in part, because of the large number of exposed nerve endings and, in part, because of the very traditional way that many donor sites are managed. Initially, a donor site is a raw haemorrhagic area. Pressure is needed to stop the bleeding and the wound should be checked regularly in the immediate postoperative period. Analgesia is also necessary and may be needed for several days.

Traditionally, donor sites have been dressed with paraffin gauze, covered with ordinary gauze, wrapped in wool roll or gamgee and held in place with bandages (Wilkinson, 1997). The dressing is left in place for about ten days and then removed. This is often a very painful experience as the dressing has dried out and adhered to the wound. The patient may have to sit in the bath in order to soak the dressing off. Damage to the newly formed tissue can occur as the dressing is pulled away. The newly epithelialising wound may be quite sore and dessicated. Aqueous cream or a similar emollient may be applied as a moisturiser.

A variety of studies have demonstrated that several of the modern products could be more effective than traditional methods. The use of hydrocolloids has been studied by several researchers. Blitz *et al.* (1985) compared a hydrocolloid dressing with saline gauze. They found a significantly faster healing time with the hydrocolloid dressing. The mean healing time was 7.2 days compared with 13.5 days with saline gauze. Pain at dressing change was also significantly less with the hydrocolloid dressing as it did not adhere to the wound. Champsaur *et al.* (1988) found similar results when comparing a hydrocolloid with paraffin gauze. They also found that the donor site was ready for re-sampling after 10 days with the hydrocolloid compared with 15 days with paraffin gauze.

Rives *et al.* (1997) found that a calcium alginate dressing significantly reduced the amount of bleeding postoperatively compared with paraffin gauze. Dressing changes were less painful in the alginate group and it was possible to reharvest from the site sooner. Although there was no significant difference in healing rates, in other aspects of care the alginate outperformed the traditional dressing. A similar study was undertaken by Reali *et al.* (1998). Each donor site acted as its own control as half the site was treated with a hydrocellular adhesive foam dressing and half with paraffin gauze. There was a significant difference in pain at dressing change. All 20 patients found the pain unbearable when the paraffin gauze was removed whereas 17 patients had no pain when the foam was removed. There was a significantly faster healing time in the foam group with 18 patients having complete epithelialisation by the fourth day.

Once the donor site has healed the skin should be kept supple. The use of emollients may be of assistance and they should be applied two or three times a day. The patient should be advised to avoid extremes of temperature. If it is not possible to avoid exposing the site to sunlight, sun blockers should be used to cover the area. Donor sites remain susceptible to sunburn. A tubular bandage may be applied to donor sites on a lower limb to provide support and to prevent hypertrophy of the scar.

Wound drains

Wound drains are inserted to provide a channel to the body surface for fluid which might otherwise collect in the wound. The fluid may be blood, pus, serous exudate, bile or other body fluids. There are several different types of drains which can be divided into open and closed drains. Open drains may be tubes, corrugated rubber or plastic, or soft tubes filled with ribbon gauze to provide a wicking effect. Open drains originally drained into the dressing, causing considerable discomfort to the patient. They also increased the risk of infection as the drain provided an open channel for bacteria. As a result of the classic research by Cruse and Foord (1973, 1980) which demonstrated the infection hazard posed by open drains they are now rarely used.

Closed drains consist of the drain, connection tubing and the collecting receptacle. They usually provide a vacuum and so have a suction effect.

Chest drains are closed drains which work rather differently. The purpose of this type of system is to allow air to escape from the chest cavity and bubble into the water in the container. Closed drains are usually inserted through a stab wound adjacent to the incision.

The use of drains is essential to prevent the collection of fluid in the wound. This is more important with some types of surgery than others. Varley and Milner (1995) randomly allocated 177 patients undergoing surgery for proximal femoral fracture to receive wound drainage or no drainage. Twice as many patients (13.2%) in the undrained group developed wound infections compared with those in the drained group (7%). However, this difference did not reach statistical significance, possibly because the numbers of infections were small. Perkins et al. (1997) randomised 222 patients undergoing face-lift surgery to drains or no drains and found a significant reduction in the formation of seromas in the group that received drainage. There was also a reduction of haematoma formation in this group, but again the difference did not reach statistical significance. Briggs (1997) reviewed several other studies looking at the use of drains in various types of surgery, in which it was found that their usage increased the risk of infection. In view of this conflicting evidence it seems reasonable to propose that drains are useful where there is a risk of haematoma formation, but that they should be removed after 24–48 hours to reduce the risk of infection.

6.2.2 Managing complications

A variety of complications may occur following surgery. Only those related to the wound will be discussed here.

Haemorrhage

Severe blood loss may occur during surgery, in the immediate postoperative period and up to ten days afterwards. This is sometimes referred to as primary, intermediary and secondary haemorrhage. The main cause of both primary and intermediary haemorrhage is poor surgical technique. This is either due to failure to control bleeding during surgery, or poorly tied blood vessels. As the blood pressure returns to normal levels the clots and ties get pushed off the end of the blood vessel(s) resulting in bleeding. Secondary haemorrhage is invariably associated with infection.

Taylor et al. (1987) studied the effects of haemorrhage on wound strength. They found that perioperative bleeding caused a weaker suture line which was associated with impaired fibroblast function. The researchers suggest that non-absorbable or long-lasting sutures should be used if haemorrhage occurs during surgery.

The bleeding may be either brisk and rapidly noticed, or more insidious. Blood may be seen on the wound dressing or it may drain into a drainage bag. If the bleeding is internal, signs of shock may be the first indication of its presence. If there is only a little bleeding, the blood may ooze into the superficial tissues and show as bruising around the suture line. Slow seeping of blood may lead to haematoma formation when the blood collects in a 'dead space' around the operative site and then clots. Plate 29 shows the drainage of a small haematoma eight days after surgery.

If there is heavy bleeding, further surgery may be needed to find and control the bleeding point. In many cases the bleeding is monitored closely to see whether further clotting will resolve the problem. When a haematoma forms it is a potential breeding ground for bacteria. It is sometimes possible to remove a suture in order to evacuate the haematoma.

Infection

Despite considerable improvement in standards of asepsis, postsurgical wound infection still occurs. In a national survey, surgical wound infection was found to account for 10.7% of all hospital-acquired infections (Emmerson et al., 1996). Measuring infection rates is one method used in evaluating standards of care for surgical audit. Overall infection rates of 4.7% (Cruse & Foord, 1980) and 7.3% (Mishriki et al., 1990) were found in surveys of the incidence of surgical wound infection. More recent surveys have tended to involve only those undergoing a particular type of surgery. For example, Noel et al. (1997) surveyed patients who had undergone clean surgery after discharge. They found an infection rate of 9% – a high rate of infection for clean wounds. They suggested that this was because they monitored patients in the community and identified infections which developed after discharge. It also emphasises the need for caution It is not possible to make direct comparisons between different surveys because of the varying methods of data collection. The criteria used for defining wound infection also vary. Crowe and Cooke (1998) have instigated a debate on case definitions of surgical wound infections and listed several definitions used by a variety of researchers. They hope that the ensuing debate will result in consensus on which definition should be used for national and international surveys.

Wilson *et al.* (1990) have addressed this problem and have produced a scoring system which they found to be reproducible. The ASEPSIS wound scoring system, with the grading for the severity of infection, is shown in Fig. 6.1. The authors compared this system with other methods when assessing 1029 surgical patients.

TABLE A

	Proportion of wound affected (%)					
Wound characteristic	0	< 20	20–29	40–59	60–79	> 80
Serous exudate	0	1	2	3	4	5
Erythema	0	1	2	3	4	5
Purulent exudate	0	2	4	6	8	10
Separation of deep tissues	0	2	4	6	8	10

TABLE B

Criteria for allocation of additional points to ASEPSIS Score	
Criterion	Points
Additional treatment:	
Antibiotics	10
Drainage of pus under local anaesthetic	5
Debridement of wound (general anaesthetic)	10
Serous discharge	daily 0–5
Erythema	daily 0–5
Purulent drainage	daily 0–10
Separation of deep tissues	daily 0–10
Isolation of bacteria	10
Stay as inpatient prolonged over 14 days	5

Score **Table A** daily for first week, add points from **Table B** for any criteria satisfied in first 2 months after surgery.

Category of infection: total score 0–10 = satisfactory healing; 11–20 = disturbance of healing; 21–30 = minor wound infection; 31–40 = moderate wound infection; > 40 = major wound infection.

Fig. 6.1 The ASEPSIS wound score. From: Wilson, A.P.R., Weavill, C., Burridge, J. & Kelsey, M.C. (1990). Reproduced with permission of Academic Press Ltd.

Further work by Wilson *et al.* (1998) reports a comparative study of four different methods of assessing wounds for infection. Patients were assessed during their hospital stay and followed up after discharge. They found that the infection rate depended on the definition being used.

When measuring the incidence of surgical wound infections it is essential to understand the potential causes. The causes of infection can be divided into factors related to the environment, the patient or the surgery, and are summarised in Table 6.1. The first two factors have already been discussed in Chapter 2. Factors relating to the surgery need to be considered, one of the most important of which is the *type* of surgery being undertaken. Cruse and Foord (1973, 1980) used a method of categorising types of surgery which has become widely recognised and used in other studies. They categorised operations into: (1) clean, (2) clean-contaminated, (3) contaminated, and (4) dirty. Table 6.2 explains these categories and shows the infection rates found by Cruse and Foord (1980). There is a quite dramatic difference in infection rates between clean and dirty surgery. The clean wound infection rate is usually used as a baseline for monitoring other factors which may affect infection rates. Richold (1992) also found different infection rates in different specialities with clean wound infection rates of 2.0% in general surgery, 2.9% in orthopaedics, 5.2% in obstetrics and 6.6% following Caesarian section.

Probably the most important factor to consider is surgical technique. Cruse and Foord (1980) found that meticulous attention to detail was essential to keep clean wound infection rates low. Mishriki *et al.* (1990) found a strong association

Table 6.1 Factors increasing the risk of surgical wound infection.

Environment

Lengthy preopertive hospitalisation
High bed occupancy
Poor standards of asepsis within the theatre suite
Unsuitable layout within the theatre suite
Inadequate ventilation in the operating theatre

Patient

Age
Obesity
Malnutrition
Diabetes
Steroids
Immunosuppressive drugs
Additional lesions e.g. pressure sore (form reservoir of bacteria)
Shaving

Wound

Type of surgery
Length of surgery
Time of surgery
Poor surgical technique
Position of drains

Based on Dealey, C. (1991).

Table 6.2 Classification of surgical wounds.

Clean
Surgery where there was no infection seen, no break in asepsis and hollow muscular organs not entered. Could include hysterectomy, cholecystectomy or appendicectomy 'in passing' if no evidence of inflammation.

Infection rate: 1.5%

Clean-contaminated
Where a hollow muscular organ is entered, but only minimal spillage of contents.

Infection rate: 7.7%

Contaminated
Where a hollow organ was opened with gross spillage of contents, acute inflammation without pus found, a major break in asepsis or traumatic wounds less than four hours old.

Infection rate: 15.2%

Dirty
Traumatic wounds more than four hours old. Surgery where a perforated viscus or pus is found.

Infection rate: 40%

Based on Cruse, P.J.E. and Foord, R. (1980).

between the individual surgeon and the development of infection. The elimination of one surgeon's case-load would have reduced the clean wound infection rate by over 40%. Mishriki *et al.* suggest that in-house surgical audit and peer review should be a fundamental aspect of quality assurance. Israelsson (1998) surveyed 1013 patients who underwent a midline laparotomy. He found the individual surgeon's infection rates ranged from 0% to 27%. Reilly (1997) audited the infection rates within a district general hospital and found a direct correlation between the grade of surgeon and infection rates; the more junior the doctor the poorer the technique was likely to be.

Other factors which have been shown to have some relevance to the development of infection includes the length of operations. Cruse and Foord (1980) found that the clean wound infection rate doubled for every hour of surgery. They suggest four possible reasons for this increase: (1) wound cells are damaged by drying out when exposed to air; (2) the total amount of bacterial contamination increases with time; (3) the longer the operation, the more sutures and electrocoagulation are used; (4) longer surgery may be associated with shock and/or blood loss, thus reducing resistance to infection. Although it is not possible to eliminate all these factors, the numbers of bacteria in the air can be reduced. Although air filtration systems can be used, Cruse and Foord suggested that the same results could be obtained by taking some fairly simple measures such as: reducing conversation and the amount of movement in and out of the theatre and excluding anyone with a skin infection.

The timing of surgery also affects infection rates. Cruse and Foord (1980) found that when clean or clean-contaminated surgery was carried out at night-time there was almost double the infection rate of that in the day. This is most likely to be due to weariness in the surgical team leading to imperfect surgical technique.

● *Nursing care* ●

Early identification of signs of infection is important. The care of infected wounds has been described in Chapter 3.

Dehiscence

Dehiscence means the breaking down, or splitting open, of all or part of a wound healing by first intention. It is most frequently seen in abdominal wounds (Westaby, 1985). Complete dehiscence may involve evisceration of the gut, a condition which is commonly known as a 'burst abdomen'. If the skin remains intact when the muscle and fascia layers break down, an incisional hernia occurs. It may not become obvious until some months following surgery.

Dehiscence can occur because of systemic and local factors. Several studies have looked at the effect of surgical wound closure techniques. Gislason *et al.* (1995) randomised 599 patients to three different types of closure. They found that there was no difference between the groups. Dehiscence occurred more frequently in those undergoing emergency surgery, those having intestinal resections with stoma formation and those with wound infections. Those patients whose wounds broke down were also significantly older. Brolin (1996) found that a continuous suture was more effective for closing midline incisions following surgery for morbid obesity than an interrupted suturing technique.

Westaby (1985) considers that surgical technique may be a factor in dehiscence. Securing sutures too tightly so that the sutures cut into the tissues can result in dehiscence. Tight suturing also affects the vascularity of the skin edges, with areas of necrosis around the sutures. Occasionally failure of the suture material may occur. This is less common with non-absorbable sutures. Perkins (1992) suggests that dehiscence can be divided into early wound dehiscence and late wound dehiscence. She suggests that early dehiscence is related to suture failure and/or surgical technique and that late dehiscence is more likely to be the result of infection.

● *Nursing care* ●

If a surgical wound starts to break down, the potential cause(s) should be identified and rectified where possible. The wound should be carefully assessed for indications of infection. If major dehiscence, such as a burst abdomen, occurs, the wound will need resuturing. Most wounds are treated conservatively and allowed to heal by granulation and contraction. This is particularly so when infection is present as all purulent material needs to be allowed free drainage.

The wounds may be necrotic or sloughy with a heavy exudate. Cannavo *et al.* (1998) compared three dressing regimes: an alginate; Eusol-soaked gauze; and a combine pad for 36 patients with dehiscent abdominal wounds. Unfortunately the numbers were too small to detect any statistical difference in healing rates. However, the patients with the Eusol soaks had a significantly higher level of wound pain. Patients were also less satisfied with this dressing compared with the other two. Costings of the three dressing regimes found that the Eusol soaks were considerably higher than the other dressings because of the greater amount of nursing time required for dressing changes.

If there is only a partial dehiscence of the suture line with little exudate and necrosis as shown in Plate 30, then an amorphous hydrogel is appropriate. This causes far less trauma than using traditional methods such as ribbon gauze. Once any cavity is filled with granulation tissue and there is no indication of lingering infection, foam cavity fillers may also be used.

In a few instances the exudate may be excessive and not controlled by dressings. In this situation it may be helpful to consult the stoma nurse, who may suggest that an appliance similar to a drainage bag be used. It has an adhesive backing which can be cut to fit over the wound, whilst protecting the surrounding skin. The front of the appliance has a hinged lid which allows access to the wound and saves frequent removal. There is usually a tap which allows drainage. The amount of exudate can be measured accurately which is important for fluid balance. Good wound management of a wound following dehiscence should promote healing and permit the patient to be discharged home for care in the community.

Sinus formation

A sinus is a track to the body surface from an abscess or some material which is an irritant and becomes a focus for infection. A common irritant is suture material. Dressing material, such as ribbon gauze may also be retained and prevent healing. Sinuses can become chronic if the causative factor is not resolved. A sinogram will show the extent of a sinus and help to identify the root problem. Surgical excision or laying open of the sinus is usually the most effective form of management. Once the focus for infection has been removed and free drainage can occur, the remaining cavity will heal by granulation and contraction.

Although wide excision is the most appropriate method of managing a sinus, it is not always possible. If the sinus is very deep the opening may be fairly narrow in relation to the sinus size. Everett (1985) suggests that inserting a drainage tube into the sinus will prevent the sinus closing and allow free drainage. The tube can gradually be withdrawn as the sinus heals.

Fistula formation

A fistula is an abnormal track connecting one viscus with another viscus or a viscus with the body surface. Fistulae develop spontaneously or following surgery. Common examples are: rectovaginal – connecting the rectum and vagina; biliary – allowing leakage of bile to the surface following surgery on the gall bladder and/or bile ducts; faecal – allowing leakage of faecal fluid through the wound, often associated with infection. Persistent leakage of fluid indicates the possible presence of a fistula. Examination of the fluid will usually provide information to indicate the source of the fistula. Any associated infection must also be treated.

● *Nursing care* ●

The management of fistulae involves care of the surrounding skin, containing and measuring the output and nutritional support. The skin can be protected by the use of ostomy pastes and protective skin wafers. Drainage bags can be applied to collect the output from the fistula. The stoma nurse may have the greatest skill in applying a suitable drainage bag over the fistula and protecting the skin.

Occasionally, it is not possible to retain a drainage bag over a fistula. In these circumstances a suction tube can be inserted by the medical staff and attached to a low-pressure suction machine. There is likely to be some leakage around the tube. The skin should be covered with protective wafer and a dressing applied to absorb the fluid.

Once the output from the fistula is contained it can be accurately measured. This enables the correct amount of fluid to be given to replace what has been lost. Output may be considerable – sometimes as much as a litre a day. In hospitals where there is a nutrition team, they can also be involved in the care of these patients. When it is possible, enteral feeding should be given. If the fistula is high in the gastrointestinal tract then it will be necessary to give parenteral nutrition.

Management of fistulae requires skilled nursing care. Several authors have described this care by means of case studies, (Pringle, 1995, Wiltshire, 1996; Beitz & Caldwell, 1998). Although some fistulae may resolve spontaneously, others will require surgical intervention. For this latter group, nursing care can only be seen to contain the problem, not resolve it.

● *Evaluation* ●

Regular monitoring of surgical wounds is essential in order to identify any potential complications. Early intervention may prevent further problems.

6.3 TRAUMATIC WOUNDS

Traumatic injuries can range from a simple cut to a major crushing injury. Major traumatic injury is beyond the remit of this book. It requires surgical intervention and specialised nursing care. Most nurses will be required to care for minor traumatic wounds from time to time.

6.3.1 Minor traumatic wounds

● *Assessment* ●

Initial assessment should be to identify any life-threatening problems, such as airway obstruction, haemorrhage or shock. Vital signs should be recorded. Any of these problems should be addressed before treating the wound.

If possible, a history should be obtained of when, where and how the injury occurred. A medical history can highlight any factors which may affect healing of the wound; this information may affect the type of treatment prescribed to manage the wound.

The wound should be assessed for any bleeding. Haemorrhage may be resolved by pressure or require surgical intervention. The presence of any foreign bodies should be noted and also the extent and severity of the injury. Cleansing of the wound may be necessary before a full assessment can be made. Loose particles may be washed off by using a 'soapy' cleanser such as Savlon®. Some accident and emergency departments use cling film to cover a wound until seen by the doctor. This has the advantage of keeping the wound warm and moist and allowing easy observation.

● *Nursing intervention* ●

Medical assessment and prescription may be necessary before the wound can be dressed. Although many nurses are competent to dress minor injuries the following guidelines should be considered.

Patients should be examined by a doctor if:

- they present at an accident and emergency department
- the nature and extent of the injury is uncertain
- there is persistent bleeding
- suturing is required
- a foreign body is present
- tetanus prophylaxis may be necessary
- the injury occurred to a hospital patient
- the nurse is uncertain of the appropriate management
- it is required by nursing policies.

Prior to dressing, the wound should be thoroughly cleaned using saline. Any loose devitalised tissue should be removed. In some instances it may be necessary to shave the area around the wound if there are hairs which may interfere with the healing process. An appropriate dressing can then be applied. Tetanus prophylaxis will be required if the patient has not had a complete course of tetanus toxoid or if no booster dose has been given for more than five years. Depending on the cause of the wound, the doctor may also prescribe a course of antibiotics.

If the patient is not a patient in hospital, then information should be provided about the management of the wound and who to contact if any complication occurs. Potential complications such as fever, swelling around the wound, excessive pain or offensive discharge should be described to the patient. Ideally, this information should also be available in written form so that the patient has it for future reference.

Traumatic injuries occur primarily to the young and the elderly. Whilst most young people will heal easily, this is not necessarily true for older people. They may need to be admitted to hospital for further care. Wijetunge (1992) has provided a useful overview of a management plan for soft tissue injuries.

● *Evaluation* ●

The aim of any treatment is uncomplicated healing of the wound with restoration of function and minimal scarring (Brunner & Suddarth, 1988). Evaluation of minor traumatic wounds may be carried out by those making the original assessment, or the patient may be referred to the family practitioner. The majority of these wounds will heal without complication.

6.3.2 The management of specific types of traumatic wounds

Abrasions

An abrasion is a superficial injury where the skin is rubbed or torn. It can be caused by falling on a gritty surface, and may be extremely sore. Abrasions should be cleaned carefully to ensure that there are no foreign bodies embedded in the wound. In the case of extensive abrasions a general anaesthetic may be required in order to allow adequate cleansing. Failure to remove all the debris may result in unsightly 'tattooing' (Evans & Jones, 1996).

Selection of a suitable dressing depends on the extent and depth of the injury. These wounds are often very sore. Occlusive dressings have been found to reduce the pain, possibly because they keep the nerve endings from drying out. If the abrasion is superficial a film dressing or a thin hydrocolloid can be applied. Deeper wounds with a heavier exudate can be covered by hydrocolloids, foams or alginates.

Lacerations

A laceration is a wound that penetrates the skin and has a torn and jagged edge. Lacerations can be caused by blunt injury which produces shear forces or by a sharp object such as glass (Singer et al., 1997). Plate 31 shows a skin tear and associated bruising in an elderly patient with very fragile skin. This injury was caused by a carer grabbing the patient's arm to prevent her falling. The aim of treatment for lacerations is to achieve uncomplicated healing with a functional and cosmetically acceptable scar.

It is important to remove all debris and any devitalised tissue from the wound. This procedure is sometimes called surgical toilet. The best way to manage lacerations is to bring the skin edges together to heal by first intention. This may be achieved by the use of sutures, adhesive strips or tissue adhesive. The choice of material depends on the position of the wound, its extent and the condition of the damaged skin. Suturing is recommended around joints or on the hand where movement is involved. Quinn et al. (1997) randomised patients with lacerations on the face, torso or extremities, excluding those involving joints, hands or feet, to either tissue adhesive or suturing. They found no difference in healing rate, but the adhesive was faster to apply and caused less pain. It also does not require removal. It is potentially a cost-effective method of treating simple lacerations.

One of the commonest positions for a laceration is the pretibial area (see Plate 32). If this injury was inflicted on a young person with healthy skin, sutures or adhesive strips would probably be used. Sutures would cause tearing in the same injury in an elderly person with fragile skin. In such circumstances, adhesive strips or glue would be more suitable. Plate 33 shows a pretibial laceration with the skin edges taped together. Healing may be promoted in an elderly person by resting and elevating the affected leg.

If there is any risk of infection as a result of severe contamination of the wound at the time of injury, primary closure is not appropriate. Conservative treatment of antibiotics and the use of dressings such as an amorphous hydrogel is preferable.

An iodine-impregnated low-adherent dressing may also be used for a short period of time. Once there is no likelihood of infection the use of a hydrogel or hydrocolloid is more suitable.

Fingertip injuries

Crushing fingertip injuries are very common in children. They are mainly caused by fingers being caught in house or car doors. Buckles (1985) suggests that 14% of children below the age of 13 years suffer from this type of injury. Cockerill and Sweet (1993) describe the procedure of trephining to remove a haematoma from the nail bed. They also suggest that an X-ray may be necessary to identify any fracture. In those circumstances, prophylactic antibiotics may be needed.

The use of adhesive tapes over the finger tip can be an effective way of holding the wound edges together. The finger can then be protected by a tubular bandage. Collier (1996) suggests that it is important to use dressings that will not adhere to the wound as adherent dressings will cause pain and further trauma at dressing change. Given that many of the patients are children, this is an important consideration. Suitable dressings might be hydrocolloids or adhesive foams which can be retained without bulky dressings or strapping.

Animal bites

Patients with animal bites frequently present in accident and emergency departments. Lewis and Styles (1995) calculated that two million patients are treated each year in the USA for bites at a cost of some $30 million. As many as 74% of bites are from dogs; other animals which cause problems include cats, rats, squirrels and, occasionally, snakes. As well as animal bites, patients also present with human bites, usually as a result of physical violence such as a punch to the mouth which results in injury to the knuckles (Higgins *et al.*, 1997).

The major problem with any type of bite injury is the risk of infection, or the transmission of diseases such as HIV or hepatitis B from human bites. Higgins *et al.* (1997) stress the importance of not underestimating these wounds. However, prophylactic antibiotics are not necessary for all patients as infections will only occur in a small number of cases (Cummings, 1994).

Careful cleansing is essential in order to assess the extent of the injury. Saline or an antimicrobial such as povidone-iodine should be used. Surgical debridement or exploration may be necessary to remove devitalised tissue, skin tags or any foreign bodies. Large cuts and facial wounds need suturing. Puncture wounds should be left open because of the risk of infection. The wound should be protected. An iodine-impregnated low-adherent dressing may be suitable, unless there is a moderate to heavy exudate.

Higgins *et al.* (1997) suggest that patients with human puncture wounds should be admitted for surgical exploration and irrigation. So, too, should those with bites involving joints or tendons or any indication of spreading infection. Patients with bite wounds should be followed up to ensure that there has been uncomplicated healing and the patient has regained full function of the affected area.

6.4 THE BURN INJURY

Burns are traumatic wounds, but because of the specialised care required, they need to be considered separately from other traumatic wounds. Generally, adults with more than 15% burns or children with more than 10% burns are treated in specialised burns units. In addition, patients with deep burns of a smaller surface area or on parts of the body such as the face may also be admitted to a burns unit. Patients with less serious burns may be cared for in any area, although in some areas they may also be taken to specialised units. An extensive description of burn care is beyond the remit of this book.

6.4.1 Aetiology

A burn is an injury caused by excessive heat. It primarily damages the skin, causing tissue destruction and coagulation of the blood vessels of the affected area. Burns are also often surrounded by an area of erythema.

Burns can be divided into four categories:

Thermal These are caused by flame, hot water or steam, other hot liquids, and hot surfaces. Smoke inhalation injuries may be associated with fire casualties.
Chemical Caused by spillage of strong acids, alkalis or other corrosive substances, these are usually industrial injuries. Damage to vital organs can occur if the chemicals are absorbed into the blood supply.
Electrical These are caused by an electrical current passing through the body. The internal damage may be considerably greater than is obvious from the skin appearance. Such burns may also be associated with thermal injury.
Radiation Radiation burns are due to overexposure to industrial ionising radiation or following radiotherapy treatment. (Reactions to radiotherapy are covered in more detail in Section 6.5.)

Although burn injuries are usually described as accidental, it has been suggested that some individuals are more likely to suffer from them than others. This has been summarised by Boore *et al.* (1987) who divided the predisposing factors into personal and environmental.

Personal factors include:

Age Children under school age are the most likely sufferers, but the very old are also vulnerable.
Sex In the under-65-years age group, more males than females have suffered burns.
Physical disability Individuals suffering from obesity, epilepsy or neurological and cardiovascular disease resulting in some degree of physical disability are vulnerable.
Psychiatric problems Individuals with a variety of problems such as alcohol or drug abuse, behavioural difficulties, a history of suicide attempts or self-destructive behaviour or a known psychiatric condition are more vulnerable.

Environmental factors include:

Family stress   Major life events resulting in stress such as moving house, social isolation, family conflicts, financial difficulties or other stressors may be found to be present at the time of injury.

Socioeconomic factors   There is an increased risk to all family members when they live in poor, overcrowded accommodation, particularly when there is unemployment or the wage earner has an unskilled or semiskilled job.

6.4.2 Incidence

Wilkinson (1998) reviewed the numbers of people in four counties in England presenting to accident and emergency departments with burns during the year 1994–95. He found that burns comprised 1% of the workload. The rate of admission was 0.14 per 1000 population per year. Children under five years of age had the highest admission rate. Lawrence (1992) suggests that one child in every 140 under school age will be admitted to hospital with thermal injury. Many of these will be scalds. Scalds are 40 times more common in children than adults. Lawrence (1992) also noted that 40% of injuries from scalds are related to tea making, if kettle scalds are included.

Staff should be aware of the possibility of non-accidental injury to children. Gordon and Goodwin (1997) suggest that around 10% of paediatric burns are the result of child abuse. This is supported by work by Andronicus *et al.* (1998). They reviewed 507 paediatric burn cases. They found that 8% of injuries were considered to be as a result of abuse or neglect. The staff believed that the family's social or emotional situation was likely to have been a major factor in causing the burn injury of a further 6% of children. Andronicus *et al.* (1998) provide a list of features that may indicate abuse or neglect. They include a delay between the incident and presentation, an inconsistent history of events, a history of previous accidents and presentation for treatment by someone other than the parent. Most accident and emergency departments have specific procedures to follow in the event of an injury being suspected to be non-accidental.

6.4.3 The severity of the injury

The skin is the organ of the body which usually suffers the greatest damage from a burn injury. Depending on the extent of the injury, several layers may be affected. It is common to describe the severity of a burn according to its depth and extent. Burns are divided into superficial, partial-thickness and full-thickness according to depth.

Superficial burns   Only the upper strata of the epithelium are damaged. The stratum basale is unaffected.

Partial-thickness burns   These burns extend beyond the epidermis into the dermis.

Full-thickness burns   There is full destruction of the epidermis and dermis. The damage extends into the subcuticular layer and may involve muscle and bone.

The extent of the burn is determined by the measurement of the surface area of the affected part, excluding erythema. This is described in terms of a percentage of the whole body. Various methods of achieving this have been described. An *ad hoc* method is to measure the area using the palm of the hand. The palmar surface of the patient is equal to 1% of the body surface area in adults and 1.5% in children. When making the initial assessment of a burn injured patient, it is most common to use the 'Rule of Nines' (Wallace, 1951). Figure 6.2 shows how the body is divided into sections, each measuring 9% of the whole, or multiples of 9%. The percentages for each affected area are then totalled. Thus, if one arm and the front of the trunk were affected, this would be described as 27% burns.

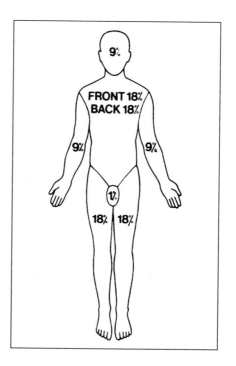

Fig. 6.2 The 'Rule of Nines'.

However, the Rule of Nines may overestimate the extent of the injury. Once the initial emergency treatment has been carried out, a reassessment of the extent of the injury is usually made. A more accurate picture can be obtained using a Lund and Browder chart (see Fig. 6.3). Lund and Browder (1944) developed a system for assessing burn injury which not only divides the body into smaller areas, but also considers the age of the patient. Body proportions alter during childhood, so that the front of the head is 8.5% of the whole in a child of one year, but only 4.5% of the whole in a 15-year-old child. Patient management may need to be adapted once this reassessment has been made.

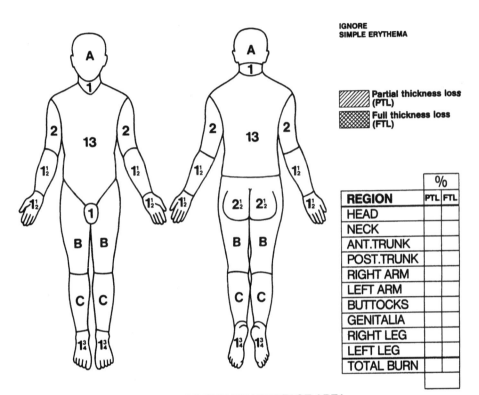

CHART FOR ESTIMATING SEVERITY OF BURN WOUND

NAME_____WARD_____NUMBER_____DATE_____
AGE_____ ADMISSION WEIGHT_____

LUND AND BROWDER CHARTS

IGNORE
SIMPLE ERYTHEMA

Partial thickness loss (PTL)

Full thickness loss (FTL)

REGION	%	
	PTL	FTL
HEAD		
NECK		
ANT.TRUNK		
POST.TRUNK		
RIGHT ARM		
LEFT ARM		
BUTTOCKS		
GENITALIA		
RIGHT LEG		
LEFT LEG		
TOTAL BURN		

RELATIVE PERCENTAGE OF BODY SURFACE AREA
AFFECTED BY GROWTH

AREA	AGE 0	1	5	10	15	ADULT
A=½ OF HEAD	9½	8½	6½	5½	4½	3½
B=½ OF ONE THIGH	2¾	3¼	4	4½	4½	4¾
C=½ OF ONE LEG	2½	2½	2¾	3	3¼	3½

Fig. 6.3 The Lund and Browder chart.

6.4.4 Burn oedema

Almost immediately after injury, oedema starts to collect beneath the damaged tissue. This is typically maximal within 24 hours of the injury, but may last for up to three or four days. As plasma continues to leak into the tissues, there is a risk of hypovolaemia developing. Without treatment, burns shock can develop and is potentially fatal. If the burn is on the face, neck or chest, the swelling from the oedema may cause obstruction of the airway. Patients with facial burns are admitted for 24 hours as a precaution. Treatment must ensure that the effects of burn oedema are minimised.

6.4.5 First-aid treatment of burns

The British Burn Association has published recommendations for the first-aid treatment of burns (Lawrence, 1987). Table 6.3 is based on these recommendations. The principal treatment is to remove the injured person from the source of heat and pour cold water over the affected area. Lawrence and Wilkins (1986) demonstrated that the subcutaneous temperature continues to rise after the burn injury occurs. Thus, if a burn injury at 100°C lasts for 10 seconds, the affected tissue will take 3 minutes to return to normal body temperature. Application of cold water within 10 seconds of the injury can reduce the 'burn time' to 30 seconds. Lawrence calls upon all healthcare workers, emergency service personnel and first aiders to publicise this treatment.

Table 6.3 The first-aid treatment of burns

- Remove the person from the source of heat.
- Turn off the electricity in the case of electrical burns.
- Apply copious amounts of water to the affected area.
- Do NOT try to remove clothing if the burns are extensive.
- Put wet compress on any exposed areas.
- Wrap cling film around wet compress to hold in place.
- Seek qualified help quickly – especially if the burn is extensive.
- If no tap water, use bottled/mineral water or milk.
- Do not use solutions such as bleach, butter or oil.

Based on Lawrence, J.C. (1987).

There are occasions when cold water is not readily available and other alternatives must be used. Lawrence (1996) tested a mousse containing a mixture of paraffin oils and waxes in the laboratory and found that it gave local cooling for at least 10 minutes. The same product was tested at a Fire Service College on 108 casualties with a variety of burns or scalds (Dunn, 1996). All subjects found immediate pain relief after application of the mousse. When the mousse fell off a thin film remained over the burn site obviating the need for a dressing unless there was skin loss. This product would appear to be a useful first-aid treatment, however, further clinical evidence is required to support its use.

6.4.6 The management of burn injuries

When considering the management of burns, the extent of the injury must be defined because the treatment varies drastically between major and minor burns.

Minor burns may be treated in the outpatient department, but anyone with major burns must be admitted to hospital. Gowar and Lawrence (1995) listed the criteria for hospital admission. These are:

(1)   Burns greater than 5% of total body area.
(2)   Burns on important areas such as face, hands, feet, perineum, joints or flexor surfaces.
(3)   History of smoke inhalation or noxious vapour or electric shock.
(4)   Patients with medical conditions such as diabetes or epilepsy.
(5)   Elderly patients, those living alone or those whose injury would limit their ability to care for themselves.
(6)   Small full-thickness burns.
(7)   Patients with any indications of wound infection or evidence of septicaemia.
(8)   Any uncertainty in relation to the cause (i.e. non-accidental) or the extent of the injury.

Major burns

Gordon and Goodwin (1997) describe the importance of the primary assessment of the patient which includes the ABCDEF assessment:

- *A = airway, B = breathing*   Check airway. Endotracheal intubation may be needed if there are deep burns to face, neck or mouth or any indication of respiratory distress.

- *C = circulation*   Check pulse. This may be absent or show signs of dysrythmias following an electrical burn.

- *D = Disability or neurological deficit*   Identify any associated trauma. Signs of mental confusion or disorientation may be an indication of pre-existing conditions, hypoxia or unrecognised injury.

- *E = exposure and evaluation*   All jewellery or clothes should be removed from the burn injured area because of the risk of constriction when burn oedema develops. This also allows for a rapid assessment of the full extent of the injury, using the Rule of Nines. The patient should be kept warm – a space blanket is ideal.

- *F = fluid resuscitation*   Establish an intravenous infusion. This is essential for all burns greater than 15% of total body surface in adults and 10% in children. Blood samples may be taken at the same time. Catheterise the bladder if the burns are 25% or more of body total; urinary output will indicate inadequate rehydration as well as renal function.

It is also important to obtain a full history of cause of the injury from patient, relative or ambulance crew. This may provide information indicating potential complications such as smoke inhalation. Analgesia, either inhalational or systemic, may be given depending on the condition of the patient.

Management of major burns is best carried out in a burns unit. If the injury occurs some considerable distance from a specialised unit, the patient may be taken first to a nearby accident and emergency department. When the patient's condition has been stabilised by the above measures, urgent transfer can take place. Once in the care of a burns team a more detailed assessment of the patient and the extent of the burn injury using a Lund and Browder chart is undertaken. If there are circumferential burns on any part of the body, it may be necessary to perform escharotomy. As burn oedema forms the burned skin is unable to stretch and thus it has a tourniquet effect. An escharotomy is a deep longitudinal incision which releases the tension.

Minor burns

Managing minor burns requires assessment of both the patient and the wound as in any other type of wound. Assessment of the patient has been discussed in Chapter 2 and wound assessment and management in Chapter 3. Specific aspects of the care of minor burns are discussed here.

● *Patient assessment* ●

Maintaining a safe environment   Discover the cause of the injury. Non-accidental injury must be considered if the history seems inconsistent with the burn appearance. The risk of infection is always present in the burn injured patient.

Communicating   It is important to provide reassurance and explanation to the patient and the family. Analgesia may be required for pain.

Eating and drinking   Nutritional status should be identified. Advice on nutrition may be necessary as there will be increased nutritional demands on the body.

Mobilising   The burn injury may affect mobility. Simple exercises may be necessary.

Expressing sexuality   A burn injury can be extremely disfiguring. Body image may be profoundly altered causing distress and loss of self-esteem.

Sleeping   Pain or anxiety may affect sleep patterns.

Psychological care   Many patients will be very frightened. Specific fears should be identified and addressed. They may be fears of disfigurement or disability. Some may fear loss of loved ones as a result of the scarring.

● *Wound assessment* ●

Initial assessment of a burn injury includes the extent and depth of the burn. The use of a Lund and Browder chart has already been described. Most burns are surrounded by an area of erythema which should not be included when calculating the burn area. Identifying the depth of a burn may not be easy. A burn injury may have varying depths. However, these guidelines may be followed:

Superficial burns

The skin looks red and dry, possibly with some oedema

Assessment	Rationale
Pin-prick test	Pain indicates undamaged nerve endings.
Light pressure which is then released	Blanching followed by refilling of capillaries indicates undamaged blood supply.

Partial-thickness burns

In shallower partial-thickness burns, the epithelium forming the shafts of the hair follicles is still intact. However, the capillary network is damaged, releasing a serous exudate which forms blisters. Beneath the blister, the wound surface appears wet, swollen and pink. Nerve endings may be exposed and the patient may experience acute pain. Deep partial-thickness burns are firmer. As more blood vessels have been destroyed, there is less exudate and blistering. The colour may vary from a waxy white to a dark red.

Assessment	Rationale
Pin-prick test	Extreme pain indicates shallow partial-thickness burn; diminished sensation indicates damaged nerve endings and a deep dermal burn.
Light pressure which is then released	Indicates the degree of damage to the capillaries, the deeper the burn, the slower the refill.
The degree of blistering and exudate	The shallower the burn, the more exudate and blisters.

Full-thickness burns

The skin often looks quite leathery and dry. The colour can be black, dark brown, tan, red or white.

Assessment	Rationale
Pin-prick test	No sensation as nerve endings are destroyed.
Burn feels hard and dry	Due to coagulation of fluid in tissues.

A burn injury differs from other types of wounds in several important respects (Bayley, 1990). There are frequently large areas of devitalised tissue. The wound may have a large surface area and take some time to heal. As a result, the burn wound is rapidly colonised by bacteria. There is considerable risk of infection in major burns, but it is much less likely in minor burns. Lawrence (1989) quotes an incidence of about 1% but this may vary between centres. Nonetheless, the wound should be observed carefully for any indication of infection.

● *Wound management* ●

The main goals in the management of burns are as follows:

- To debride burn eschar, if present.
- To promote rapid healing.
- To prevent/detect infection.

Debridement of burn eschar can be achieved by surgical debridement or by using a dressing which will promote the autolytic processes of the body. Selection of the method will depend on the burn appearance and possibly the age of the patient. Surgical debridement would certainly be inappropriate in a frightened child who resisted all attempts to be held still.

The product which has been used most widely on burns is silver sulphadiazine. It is the dressing of choice for major burns until grafting can take place. Silver sulphadiazine has an antimicrobial effect and is effective against Gram-negative and *Candida* sp. It thus has the advantage of helping to prevent infection. However, high standards of asepsis are still required at dressing change.

In minor burns, other types of wound management products are also used. Small partial-thickness burns have traditionally been treated with an antiseptic-impregnated tulle, or paraffin gauze dressings covered with gauze and a bandage. Although healing will occur with this regime, there are several disadvantages: the dressings are bulky and hinder washing around the affected area; they may also be painful to remove, although it may not be necessary to remove the wound contact layer until the wound is healed and it separates spontaneously.

Hydrocolloids may be used and can absorb exudate. Thomas *et al.* (1995) undertook a randomised study comparing a hydrocolloid alone, a hydrocolloid with silver sulphadiazine cream, and a medicated paraffin gauze dressing in 50 patients with 54 minor burns. The hydrocolloid group required significantly fewer dressings than the other two groups. The hydrocolloid group also had significantly faster healing than the hydrocolloid with cream group. The researchers concluded that hydrocolloid dressings alone can be useful for the management of minor burns.

Other dressings that can be used on minor burns include flat foam dressings and hydrogels. The foam dressings are comfortable and can be held in place with tape or a tubular net. Hydrogels can give a cooling sensation when applied which may be comforting to the patient.

Burns of the hands are best treated with silver sulphadiazine. Once the cream is applied the hand should be covered by a plastic bag. This will allow free movement and help to prevent contractures. The hand should be kept elevated for the first 48–72 hours to reduce swelling (Fowler, 1996). There are several disadvantages with the use of plastic bags. They cause considerable maceration of the whole hand as large quantities of exudate accumulate in the bag. The bag becomes heavy and pulls the wrist into flexion. Once full of fluid, the bag tends to leak or tear, necessitating dressing change. Terrill *et al.* (1991) compared the use of Gore-Tex® bags with plastic bags. Gore-Tex® has the property of water vapour permeability. Although there was no difference in healing times, there was a considerable reduction in skin maceration and accumulation of exudate when using Gore-Tex®. Improved hand function was also noted. Witchell and Crossman (1991) compared the use of these bags over silver sulphadiazine with paraffin gauze for children with burns of the hands. They found that use of Gore-Tex® bags increased child activity and reduced the length of time of dressing change. More significantly, there were considerably fewer unscheduled visits to the accident and emergency department because of problems with the dressing.

● *Evaluation* ●

Evaluation of the burns wound involves both monitoring of the wound as it progresses towards healing and of the healed wound. Once the wound is healed, special care needs to be taken of the newly formed epithelia. Bayley (1990) suggests cleansing with a mild soap and then applying water-based cream several times a day. The patient should be warned to avoid any possibility of sun burn.

Potential problems which can develop are contractures and hypertrophic scarring. Myofibroblasts contract and shorten the wound, causing the collagen fibres to become coiled. The scar develops a hard, red, raised appearance. If the burn injury is over a joint, as the myofibroblasts contract it causes flexion of the joint. Unless measures are taken to splint the joint, it will become contracted. A programme of exercise and splinting to counteract this will be established by the physiotherapist as appropriate.

Hypertrophic scarring is often managed by pressure garments which the patients will have to wear for about a year. However, a randomised study by Chang *et al.* (1995) found that pressure garments made no difference to the degree of scarring. An alternative treatment, using a silicone gel sheet, has been used, initially in Australia. Davey (1997b) has described the practice within one burns unit and illustrated the benefits by means of case studies. A randomised controlled trial is needed to determine the true efficacy of silicone gel sheets.

A few patients will develop permanent pigmentation changes. This is possibly because of damage to the melanocytes in the basal layer of the epidermis. It can present as either apigmentation or hyperpigmentation. It is not possible to predict when it will occur.

6.5 RADIATION REACTIONS

A radiation reaction is the reaction of the skin to the effects of radiotherapy and is limited to the treatment field or its exit point. Strictly speaking, a radiation reaction is not a wound. However, the skin reaction is akin to a superficial burn and has the potential for ulceration. There is insufficient research into the management of what can be a very painful problem.

6.5.1 Aetiology

Radiotherapy, using ionising radiation, is the mainstay of cancer treatment. Treatment is usually given in a series of doses, ranging from daily to weekly, although a small number of patients will receive just one dose. A course of treatment may last up to eight weeks. Radiation reactions are most likely to occur when the treatment field is close to the body surface, such as the head or neck, or if it includes axillae, under breasts, perineum or groin. The reaction is dose-dependent – that is, the more frequent the treatment or the higher the dose, the more likely the reaction. A reaction may occur during a course of treatment or after it is completed. Within six weeks of completion of treatment, all but the most severe reactions have disappeared.

6.5.2 The classification of radiation reactions

The severity of radiation reactions are generally classified at three levels (Dunne-Daly (1995), as follows:

- Erythema: the area becomes reddened and there may be some inflammation.
- Dry desquamation: the skin is red, dry, itchy and peeling.
- Wet desquamation: the skin is red and painful with blistering and weeping.

A small study of women being treated for breast cancer found that they all had skin reactions of varying degrees (Lawton & Twoomey, 1991). The worst reactions occurred within three weeks of completing treatment and lasted for several weeks. The commonest reaction was tenderness and itching. This occurred in 65% of the sample. Other reactions included tightness of skin, erythema and moist desquamation, the latter occurring in 45% of the women.

6.5.3 Management of the skin

There is considerable confusion and ritualistic practice concerning how the skin within the treatment field should be managed whilst radiotherapy is in progress (Campbell & Lane, 1996). Some centres suggest that the skin should not be washed at all during the course of treatment. Not only is this highly unacceptable to patients but there is some evidence to suggest that washing may reduce skin reactions. Campbell and Lane (1996) recommend that the area be washed according to the patient's wishes and patted dry, taking care not to remove the special markings indicating the treatment field.

There has been little research into the management of radiation reactions. However, they can be classed as a minor burn and basic principles of wound care can provide some guidelines.

(1)   All patients undergoing radiotherapy to vulnerable areas such as breast, groin or neck should apply a simple moisturiser to the area twice daily during their course of treatment.

(2)   If erythema develops the moisturiser should be applied more frequently in order to counteract the dryness of the skin.

(3)   Moisturisers can also be used for dry desquamation. Thomas (1992) found that a wide range of creams are in use, the most popular being hydrocortisone cream, but that little research has been undertaken to support any particular selection. The study by Lawton and Twoomey (1991) found that the use of a hydrocortisone cream conferred no added benefit. They suggest that Calendula cream may have a greater effect.

(4)   There is insufficient evidence to suggest a definitive treatment for wet

desquamation. The main goal is to choose a dressing that is comfortable for the patient and promotes healing. Depending on the level of exudate this could include hydrocolloids, hydrogels and foams.

6.5.4 Care of the patient

The most important aspect of care of any patient undergoing radiotherapy must be communication. Frith (1991) has reviewed the literature on information related to radiotherapy and concluded that patients often receive little or no information prior to treatment. This results in many unmet needs. She describes the type of information that patients need, such as what side-effects to expect and how they can be managed. Written information can be used to reinforce verbal explanations. This provides the patient with a permanent record which can be shared with others.

REFERENCES

Andronicus, M., Oates, R.K., Peat, J., Spalding, S., Martin, H. (1998) Non-accidental burns in children. *Burns*, **24** (6), 552–558.

Bale, S. (1997) The evaluation of Cavi-care cavity wound dressing in the management of surgically created cavity wounds, in (eds) Leaper, D.J., Cherry, G.W., Dealey, C., Lawrence, J.C., Turner, T.D., *Proceedings of the 6th European Conference on Advances in Wound Management*. Macmillan Magazines Ltd, London.

Bayley, E.W. (1990) Wound healing in the patient with burns. *Nursing Clinics of North America*, **25** (1), 205–222.

Beitz, J.M., Caldwell, D. (1998) Abdominal wound with enterocutaneous fistula: a case study. *Journal of Wound, Ostomy and Continence Nursing*, **25** (2), 102–106.

Berry, D.P., Bale, S., Harding, K.G. (1996) Dressings for treating cavity wounds. *Journal of Wound Care*, **5** (1), 10–13.

Blitz, H., Kiessling, M., Kreysel, H.W. (1985) Comparison of hydrocolloid dressing and saline gauze in the treatment of skin graft donor sites, in (ed) Ryan, T.J., *An Environment for Healing: The Role of Occlusion*. Royal Society of Medicine, London.

Boore, J., Champion, R., Ferguson, M.C. (1987) *Nursing the Physically Ill Adult*. Churchill Livingstone, Edinburgh.

Briggs, M. (1996) Surgical wound pain: a trial of two treatments. *Journal of Wound Care*, **5** (10), 456–460.

Briggs, M. (1997) Principles of closed surgical wound care. *Journal of Wound Care*, **6** (6), 288–292.

Brolin, R.E. (1996) Prospective, randomised evaluation of midline fascial closure in gastric bariatric operations. *American Journal of Surgery*, **172**, 328–331.

Brunner, L.S., Suddarth, D.S. (1988) *Textbook of Medical-Surgical Nursing*. J.B. Lippincott Company, Philadelphia.

Buckles, E. (1985) Wound care in accident and emergency. *Nursing*, **2** (42 Suppl.), 3–5.

Campbell, J., Lane, C. (1996) Developing a skin-care protocol in radiotherapy. *Professional Nurse*, **12** (2), 105–108.

Cannavo, M., Fairbrother, G., Owen, D., Ingle, J., Lumley, T. (1998) A comparison of dressings in the management of surgical abdominal wounds. *Journal of Wound Care*, **7** (2), 57–62.

Champsaur, A., Amadou, R., Nefzi, A., Marichy, J. (1988) Use of Duoderm on donor sites after skin grafting. A comparative study with tulle-gras, in (ed) Ryan, T.J., *Beyond Occlusion: Wound Care Proceedings*. Royal Society of Medicine, London.

Chang, P., Laubenthal, K.N., Lewis, R.W. II, Rosenquist, M.D., Lindley-Smith, P. Kealey, G.P. (1995) A prospective randomised study of the efficacy of pressure garment therapy in patients with burns. *Journal of Burn Care Rehabilitation*, **16**, 473–475.

Chrintz, H., Vibits, H., Harreby, J.S., Cordtz, T.O., Waadegaard, P., Larsen, S.O. (1989) Need for surgical wound dressing. *British Journal of Surgery*, **76**, 204–205.

Cockerill, J., Sweet, A. (1993) Nursing management of common accident wounds. *British Journal of Nursing*, **2** (11), 578–582.

Collier, M. (1996) Trauma injury nursing in A & E. *Nursing Times*, **93** (20), 74–79.

Coull, A., Wylie, K. (1990) Regular monitoring: the way to ensure flap healing. *Professional Nurse*, **6** (1), 18–21.

Crowe, M.J., Cooke, E.M. (1998) Review of case definitions for nosocomial infection – towards consensus. *Journal of Hospital Infection*, **39**, 3–11.

Cruse, P.J.E., Foord, R. (1973) A five-year prospective study of 23,649 surgical wounds. *Archives of Surgery*, **107**, 206–210.

Cruse, P.J.E., Foord, R. (1980) The epidemiology of wound infection, a ten-year prospective study of 62,939 wounds. *Surgical Clinics of North America*, **60** (1), 27–40.

Cummings, P. (1994) Antibiotics to prevent infection in patients with dog bites: a meta-analysis of randomised trials. *Annals of Emergency Medicine*, **23** (3), 535–540.

Davey, R.B. (1997a) The use of an 'adhesive contact medium' (Hyperfix) for split skin graft fixation. *Burns*, **23** (7/8), 615–619.

Davey, R.B. (1997b) The use of contact media for burn scar hypertrophy. *Journal of Wound Care*, **6** (2), 80–82.

Dealey, C. (1991) Managing surgical wounds. *Nursing*, **4** (43), 29–32.

Dunn, R.J. (1996) Practical application of a first-aid treatment for burns and scalds. *Journal of Wound Care*, **5** (6), 265–266.

Dunne-Daly, C.F. (1995) Skin and wound care in radiation oncology. *Cancer Nursing*, **18** (2), 144–162.

Emmerson, A.M., Enstone, J.E., Griffin, M., Kelsey, M.C., Smyth, E.T. (1996) The second national prevalence survey of infection in hospitals – overview of the results. *Journal of Hospital Infection*, **32**, 175–190.

Evans, R.C., Jones, N.L. (1996) The management of abrasions and bruises. *Journal of Wound Care*, **5** (10), 465–468.

Everett, W.G. (1985) Wound sinus or fistula? in (ed) Westaby, S., *Wound Care*. William Heinemann Medical Books Ltd, London.

Foster, L., Moore, P. (1997) The application of a cellulose-based fibre dressing in surgical wounds. *Journal of Wound Care*, **6** (10), 469–473.

Fowler, A. (1996) Superficial partial-thickness burns of the hands. *Nursing Standard*, **11** (6), 56–61.

Francis, A. (1998) Nursing management of skin graft sites. *Nursing Standard*, **12** (33), 41–44.

Frith, B. (1991) Giving information to radiotherapy patients. *Nursing Standard*, **5** (34), 33–35.

Gallico, G.G., O'Connor, N.E., Compton, C.C., Kehinde, O., Green, H. (1984) Permanent cover of large burn wounds with autologous cultured human epithelium. *New England Journal of Medicine*, **311**, 448–451.

Gislason, H., Gronbech, J.E., Soreide, O. (1995) Burst abdomen and incisional hernia after major gastrointestinal operations – comparison of three closure techniques. *European Journal of Surgery*, **161**, 349–354.

Gordon, M., Goodwin, C.W. (1997) Initial assessment, management and stabilisation. *Nursing Clinics of North America*, **32** (2), 237–249.

Gowar, J.P., Lawrence, J.C. (1995) The incidence, causes and treatment of minor burns. *Journal of Wound Care*, **4** (2), 71–74.

Gupta, R., Foster, M.E., Miller, E. (1991) Calcium alginate in the management of acute surgical wounds and abscesses. *Journal of Tissue Viability*, **1** (4), 115–116.

Harding, K.G. (1990) Wound care: putting theory into clinical practice, in (ed) Krasner, D., *Chronic Wound Care*. Health Management Publications Inc., King of Prussia, Pennsylvania.

Higgins, M.A.G., Evans, R.C., Evans, R.J. (1997) Managing animal bite wounds. *Journal of Wound Care*, **6** (8), 377–380.

Holm, C., Pederson, J.S., Gronbaek, F., Gottrup, F. (1997) Occlusive versus dry wound healing: a prospective randomised study in abdominal surgery patients, in (eds) Leaper, D.J., Cherry, G.W., Dealey, C., Lawrence, J.C., Turner, T.D., *Proceedings of the 6th European Conference on Advances in Wound Management*. Macmillan Magazines Ltd, London.

Israelsson, L.A. (1998) The surgeon as a risk factor for complications of midline incisions. *European Journal of Surgery*, **164** (5), 353–359.

Lawrence, J.C. (1987) British Burn Association recommended first aid for burns and scalds. *Burns*, **13** (2), 153.

Lawrence, J.C. (1989) Treating minor burns. *Nursing Times*, **85**, 69–73.

Lawrence, J.C. (1992) The epidemiology of burns, in (eds) Harding, K.G., Leaper, D.L., Turner, T.D., *Proceedings of the 1st European Conference on Advances in Wound Management*. Macmillan Magazines Ltd, London.

Lawrence, J.C. (1996) A first-aid preparation for burns and scalds. *Journal of Wound Care*, **5** (6), 262–264.

Lawrence, J.C., Wilkins, M.D. (1986) The epidemiology of burns, in (ed) Lawrence, J.C. *Burncare*. Smith and Nephew Medical Ltd, Hull.

Lawton, J., Twoomey, M. (1991) Skin reactions to radiotherapy. *Nursing Standard*, **6** (10), 53–54.

Lewis, K.T., Styles, M. (1995) Management of dog and cat bites. *American Family Physician*, **52**, 479–485.

Lund, C.C., Browder, N.C. (1944) Estimations of areas of burns. *Surgery, Gynaecology and Obstetrics*, **79**, 352.

Marks, J., Harding, K.G., Hughes, L.E., Ribeiro, C.D. (1985) Pilonidal sinus excision healing by open granulation. *British Journal of Surgery*, **72**, 637–640.

Mishriki, S.F., Law, D.J.W., Jeffery, P.J. (1990) Factors affecting the incidence of postoperative wound infection. *Journal of Hospital Infection*, **16**, 223–230.

Noel, I., Hollyoak, V., Galloway, A. (1997) A survey of the incidence and care of postoperative wound infections in the community. *Journal of Hospital Infection*, **36**, 267–273.

Perkins, P. (1992) Wound dehiscence: causes and care. *Nursing Standard*, **6** (34 Suppl.), 12–14.

Perkins, S.W., Williams, J.D., Macdonald, K., Robinson, E.B. (1997) Prevention of seromas and haematomas after face-lift surgery with the use of postoperative vacuum drains. *Archives of Otolaryngology, Head & Neck Surgery*, **123** (7), 743–745.

Platt, A.J., Phipps, A., Judkins, K. (1996) A comparative study of silicone net dressing and paraffin gauze dressing in skin-grafted sites. *Burns*, **22** (7), 543–545.

Pringle, W. (1995) The management of patients with enterocutaneous fistulas. *Journal of Wound Care*, **4** (5), 211–213.

Quinn, J., Wells, G., Sutcliffe, T., Jarmuske, M., Maw, J., Stiell, I., Johns, P. (1997) A randomised trial comparing octylcyanoacrylate tissue adhesive and sutures in the management of lacerations. *Journal of the American Medical Association*, **277** (19), 1527–1530.

Reali, U.M., Martini, L., Borgognoni, L., Brandani, P., Andriesson, A. (1998) A hydro-cellular dressing in the treatment of partial-thickness skin graft donor sites, in (eds) Leaper, D., Cherry, G., Cockbill, S., Dealey, C., Flanagan, M., Hofman, D., *et al.*, *Proceedings of the EWMA/Journal of Wound Care Spring Meeting*. Macmillan Magazine Ltd, London.

Reilly, J. (1997) Under surveillance. *Nursing Times*, **93** (23), 57–60.

Ricci, E., Aloesio, R., Cassino, R., Ferraris, C., Gorrino, S., Anselmetti, G. (1998) Foam dressing versus gauze soaks in the treatment of surgical wounds healing by secondary intention, in (eds) Leaper, D., Cherry, G., Cockbill, S., Dealey, C., Flanagan, M., Hofman, D., *et al.*, *Proceedings of the EWMA/Journal of Wound Care Spring Meeting*. Macmillan Magazines Ltd, London.

Richold, J.C. (1992) Review of postoperative surgical wound infection in a district general hospital, in (eds) Harding, K.G., Leaper, D.L., Turner, T.D., *Proceedings of the 1st European Conference on Advances in Wound Management*. Macmillan Magazines Ltd, London.

Rives, J.M., Castede, J.C., Pannier, M., Martinot, V., Bohbot, S. (1997) Calcium alginate (Algosteril®) versus paraffin gauze in the treatment of scalp donor sites in children: results of a randomised study, in (eds) Leaper, D.J., Cherry, G.W., Dealey, C., Lawrence, J.C., Turner, T.D., *Proceedings of the 6th European Conference on Advances in Wound Management*. Macmillan Magazines Ltd, London.

Ryan, T.J. (1987) *The Management of Leg Ulcers*. Oxford University Press, Oxford.

Singer, A.J., Hollander, J.E., Quinn, J.V. (1997) Evaluation and management of traumatic lacerations. *New England Journal of Medicine*, **337** (16), 1142–1148.

Taylor, D.E.M., Whamond, J.S., Penhallow, J.E. (1987) Effects of haemorrhage on wound strength and fibroblast function. *British Journal of Surgery*, **74**, 316–319.

Terrill, P.J., Kedwards, S.M., Lawrence, J.C. (1991) The use of Gore-Tex® bags for hand burns. *Burns*, **17** (2), 161–165.

Thomas, S. (1992) *Current Practices in the Management of Fungating Lesions and Radiation-Damaged Skin*. Surgical Materials Testing Laboratory, Bridgend.

Thomas, S.S., Lawrence, J.C., Thomas, A. (1995) Evaluation of hydrocolloids and topical medication in minor burns. *Journal of Wound Care*, **4** (5), 218–220.

Varley, G.W., Milner, S.A. (1995) Wound drains in proximal femoral fracture surgery: a randomised prospective trial of 177 patients. *Journal of the Royal College of Surgeons of Edinburgh*, **40**, 416–418.

Wallace, A.B. (1951) The exposure treatment of burns. *Lancet*, **i**, 501–504.

Weiss, Y. (1983) Simplified management of operative wounds by early exposure. *International Surgery*, **68**, 237–240.

Westaby, S. (1985) Wound closure and drainage, in (ed) Westaby, S., *Wound Care*. William Heinemann Medical Books Ltd, London.

Wijetunge, D. (1992) An A & E approach. *Nursing Times*, **88** (46), 70–76.

Wilkinson, B. (1997) Hard graft. *Nursing Times*, **93** (16), 63–68.

Wilkinson, E. (1998) The epidemiology of burns in secondary care, in a population of 2.6 million people. *Burns*, **24** (2), 139–143.

Williams, P., Howells, R.E.J., Miller, E., Foster, M.E. (1995) A comparison of two alginate dressings used in surgical wounds. *Journal of Wound Care*, **4** (4), 170–172.

Wilson, A.P.R., Weavill, C., Burridge, J., Kelsey, M.C. (1990) The use of the wound scoring method 'ASEPSIS' in postoperative wound surveillance. *Journal of Hospital Infection*, **16**, 297–300.

Wilson, A.P.R., Helder, N., Theminimulle, S.K., Scott, G.M. (1998) Comparison of wound scoring methods for use in audit. *Journal of Hospital Infection*, **39**, 119–126.

Wiltshire, B.L. (1996) Challenging enterocutaneous fistula: a case presentation. *Journal of Wound, Ostomy and Continence Nursing*, **23** (6), 297–301.

Witchell, M., Crossman, C. (1991) Dressing burns in children. *Nursing Times*, **87** (36), 63–66.

Wood, R.A.B., Hughes, L.E. (1975) Silicone foam sponge for pilonidal sinus: a new technique for managing open granulating wounds. *British Medical Journal*, **3**, 131–133.

Chapter 7
Three Case Studies

7.1 INTRODUCTION

There is often discussion about the gap between theory and practice. This chapter is a series of case studies which are intended to demonstrate how the basic principles of wound care might be applied. They have been written using simple documentation rather than in full text form. The use of assessment forms provides a framework to follow and reduces the amount of writing.

NB: Examples of particular wound management products are given in these case studies. This should not be seen as an endorsement of these products compared with others; other products could be used with equally satisfactory results.

7.2 THE CARE OF A PATIENT WITH A PRESSURE SORE

Background information

Mrs Edna Turner has been admitted for rehabilitation following a stroke. She has a right-sided hemiparesis. She has a pressure sore on her right buttock.

Summary of history and patient assessment

Mrs Turner is a 76-year-old widow who lives alone in a small bungalow in a complex with a warden on call for emergencies. She has five children, all of whom are married and four families live close by. They have agreed that the eldest, Mrs Jane Reardon, will be the point of contact in the first instance. Mrs Turner is determined that she is going home and her family have said they will support her in this wish.

Communicating   Initially Mrs Turner had some slurring of her speech, but it is now improving.

Eating and drinking   Mrs Turner has lost weight recently. Her daughter says that she has not been eating properly since her husband died four months ago. Her current nutritional status is poor and she is having difficulty feeding herself.

Eliminating   Mrs Turner has had occasional episodes of incontinence which she has found very distressing.

Personal cleansing and dressing   Mrs Turner requires assistance.

Mobilising   Mrs Turner is bed- or chair-bound. She can mobilise from bed to chair with the assistance of two nurses. She has a tendency to slip to one side when sitting which is a probable factor in the development of the pressure sore on her buttock.

Psychological assessment Mrs Turner seems to be a very independent lady. She gets extremely frustrated when her body does not respond the way she wants. Her daughter says that she has been quite withdrawn since her husband died.

Spiritual assessment Mrs Turner has said several times that she wished she were dead and that she is no use to anyone.

● *Nursing assessment* ●

TISSUE VIABILITY DEPARTMENT

OPEN WOUND ASSESSMENT CHART

Type of Wound	Pressure sore Grade 3
How long has wound been open?	1 week
Location	R Buttock
General patient factors which may delay healing. (e.g. malnourished, diabetic, chronic infection, medication)	Waterlow Score 25 poorly nourished
Allergies to wound care products	None known.
Previous treatments used.	?hydrocolloid - all rolled up in bed.
Pressure Relieving Equipment (e.g. pressure relieving bed, cushion)	Autoexcel - awaiting cushion from physio.

Wound Factors	Date:	6th June 98			
Wound Classification healthy granulation epithelialisation slough black/brown necrotic tissue infected		Sloughy			
Exudate - Amount		moderate			
Odour offensive/some/none		none			
Wound Dimensions	length width depth	7 cm 5 cm 0.5 cm			
Wound Photographed?		No			
Pain (Site) at wound site elsewhere (specify)		wound "sore"			
Pain (frequency) continuous/intermittent/ only at dressing changes/ at night/none		intermittent			
Pain (severity) 0 = none 10 = excruciating		4			
Condition of surrounding skin (fragile, reddened, dry etc)		red, fragile			
Refer to CNS in Tissue Viability	Y/N Date	Yes 6th June			
Wound Assessed by:		*J. Brown*			
Next Review date:					

Multidisciplinary team communications

Effective care will require input from several members of the multidisciplinary team. The list below denotes the team members involved and their assessment of the patient.

Team member	Assessment	Outcome
Speech therapist	Swallowing assessment	No problems.
Physiotherapist	Seating assessment to give pressure relief and improved posture	Low Profile RoHo® cushion provided for wheelchair.
	General mobility assessment	Physiotherapy commenced.
Occupational therapist	Functional assessment	Assistance with washing and dressing to improve independence.
Dietitian	Nutritional assessment	High protein diet + two supplement drinks daily. Discussed with daughter, family will help with feeding meals until patient can self-care.
Hospital chaplain	Assessment for spiritual distress	Patient acknowledges that she has been 'low' since husband's death; to go to hospital chapel for special prayers before Sunday service.

● *Nursing interventions* ●

Nursing care plan

Problem	Goal	Action	Rationale	Evaluation
Pressure sore.	To promote rapid healing by 2nd intention.	(1) Clean sore by irrigation using warm saline; dry surrounding skin.	Reduces trauma to wound.	
		(2) Apply Skin-Prep® to skin round pressure sore.	Protects fragile skin.	
		(3) Apply Granuflex Bordered® 15 × 15 cm.	Encourages autolysis of slough. Border prevents dressing rolling up.	
		(4) Check dressing daily for leakage or signs of slipping, change when necessary or every 5 days.	Ensures maximum performance from dressing.	Daily.
		(5) Measure sore weekly and record on chart.	Provides objective record.	Weekly.
		(6) Place patient on Autoexcel® mattress.	Provides pressure relief.	
		(7) Turn patient 4–6 hrly when in bed.	Less disturbance of sleep.	
Date: . . . . 6 June		(8) Patient to sit out for 2 hrs 2 × daily at meal times.	Reduces pressure on pressure sore. Sitting out improves patient morale and encourages her to eat.	
Signature: . . . . J. Brown				

The outcome of care

The slough debrided from the wound rapidly and the pressure sore went on to heal without complication. Mrs Turner no longer required the alternating air overlay and had a foam pressure-reducing mattress instead. She made good progress with her rehabilitation and was ultimately discharged home.

7.3 THE CARE OF A PATIENT WITH A LEG ULCER

Background information

Mr Sidney Johnson has been referred to a nurse-led leg ulcer clinic by his GP with a leg ulcer which has deteriorated *rapidly* over the last month.

Summary of history and patient assessment

Mr Johnson is a 75-year-old retired welder; he is a widower and lives alone. He has a daughter living close by.

Eating and drinking   Mr Johson's nutritional status is reasonably good as his daughter cooks for him several times a week.
Personal cleansing and dressing   Mr Johnson is managing with difficulty, since he also suffers from arthritis quite badly in his hands.
Mobilising   Mr Johnson has limited mobility; he gets breathless sometimes and needs aids to help him walk. His daughter shops for him weekly.

● *Nursing assessment* ●

LEG ULCER ASSESSMENT FORM

NAME HOSPITAL NO. ...*Sidney JOHNSON*................................ **ADDRESS** ....*6 Blake Lane*................................... .... **TEL.NO.** .... **AGE**....*75 yrs*....... **SEX** (**M**)/ **F**	**G.P.** *Dr. Mostyn*.................... **DATE** ....*20th July*..........

Occupation (prior to retirement)   *Welder*

Height:.............................
Weight:..........................
Urine:...*N.A.D.*.................

Mobility:

Walks Independently	
Walks with aids	√
Chairbound	

Previous Medical History: please tick boxes where appropriate

M.I.			Pulmonary Embolism	
CVA/TIA			Previous DVT	
Claudication			Thrombo Phlebitis	
Prev. Arterial Surgery			Lower Leg Fractures	
Diabetes			Prev. V.V./ Surgery	
Arthritis	*hands*	√	Prev. Sclerotherapy	
Leg Oedema			Lipodermatosclerosis	
Smoker	*stopped 6/12 ago*	√	Anaemia	
Poor Nutrition			No. of pregnancies	

Other (specify)____ *"Gets a bit breathless" sometimes*_____

Record Allergies -_____ *None known*_____

Record Present Medication: ___*Co-proxamol 10 mg for pain, patient only takes it*
_____*when pain severe*_____

ULCER HISTORY

Is this the first episode of ulceration   (YES / NO)

	Right Leg	**Left Leg**
Number of Previous Episodes		
Onset of First Ulcer (years)		
Duration of Current Ulcer (months)	6/12	

Ankle Movements:

	Right Leg	Left Leg
Full	√	√
Restricted		
Fixed		

	Right Leg	Left Leg
Calf measurements (cms)	36	36
Ankle measurements (cms)	24	24.5

Doppler Reading $= \dfrac{\text{Ankle Pressure}}{\text{Brachial Pressure}}$

	Right Leg	Left Leg
Ankle Pressure	55	140
Brachial Pressure	155	155
Ankle/Brachial Pressure Index (ABPI)	.35	.9

Pain:

Continuous	☐	During Day	☐	During Night	√
At Dressing Change	☐	On mobilising	☐	None	☐

Ulcer Type - Please circle all that apply:

Venous   (Arterial)   Arthritic   Vasculitic

Diabetic   Mixed Aetiology   Traumatic   Malignancy

other ....

INITIAL ULCER ASSESSMENT

Identify ulcers by letter (A,B,C etc)

Right Leg

Width	5		
Length	9		
Shallow			
Deep (>0.2cm)	√		

Left Leg

Width			
Length			
Shallow			
Deep (>0.2cm)			

NB only measure or trace ulcers greater than 5cm diameter

Wound Traced   (YES)/ NO   **Wound Photographed**   (YES)/ NO

Wound Bed	Right Leg	Left Leg		**Exudate Levels**		Right Leg	Left Leg
Necrotic	√			High	!		
Infected				Moderate			
Sloughy	√			Low		√	
Granulating				Increasing	!		
Epithelialising				Decreasing			

! may indicate cellulitis

Wound Margin/Surrounding Skin

Macerated	☐	Oedematous	☐	Reddened	☐
Paper Thin	√	Eczema	☐	Dry/Scaling	√

Other Problems/Comments

● *Nursing interventions* ●

Treatment Plan:		Rationale:
1.	Refer for urgent vascular opinion	Probably needs surgical intervention
2.	Intrasite® & pad to ulcer	Debride - necrotic tissue
3.	Use orthopaedic wool & Tubifast® to retain dressing	No compression on arterial ulcers
4.	Simple emollient to skin	To improve dryness and loosen scales
5.	Encourage patient to take analgesia more regularly	To improve pain control

Goal:

Maintain ulcer until seen by vascular surgeon

Frequency of Evaluation: please circle

(2 / 52)   1 / 12   3 / 12

Letter to District Nurse [√]
Letter to G.P. [√]

Signature ____*J. Jones*_____

Outcome of care

Mr Johnson was seen by the vascular surgeon two weeks after his visit to clinic and underwent arterial surgery. He made an uneventful recovery and his ABPI in his right leg improved to .85. His ulcer healed within three months.

7.4 THE CARE OF A PATIENT WITH A SURGICAL WOUND

Background information

Mrs Hannah Briggs has been admitted following referral by her GP with a dehiscent wound following coronary artery bypass graft two weeks ago.

Summary of history and patient assessment

Mrs Briggs is 68 years old and lives with her husband in their own house. She was very frightened as she felt as though her chest might burst open. She said that she has been coughing a lot, but otherwise has felt quite well.

Breathing   Mrs Briggs seemed to cough quite often during assessment. She says that she is already less breathless than before the operation.

Eating and drinking   Mrs Briggs has not eaten much for the last few days but before that she was eating normally.

Eliminating   Mrs Briggs is constipated and complains of feeling uncomfortable.

Personal cleansing   Mrs Briggs is self-caring.

Psychological assessment   She is very frightened about what has happened to her wound and needs a great deal of reassurance.

Medical assessment and outcome

Mrs Briggs was found to have a chest infection and was prescribed a course of antibiotics.

Assessment by clinical nurse specialist in tissue viability and outcome

The main concern for the clinical nurse specialist was to explain exactly what had happened to Mrs Briggs and that it was only the skin layer which had failed, she still had strong metal stitches holding her chest wall together. The purpose of the dressing was also explained so that Mrs Briggs was comfortable with her care.

● *Nursing assessment* ●

TISSUE VIABILITY DEPARTMENT

OPEN WOUND ASSESSMENT CHART

Type of Wound	dehiscent surgical wound			
How long has wound been open?	2 days			
Location	mid-sternum			
General patient factors which may delay healing. (e.g. malnourished, diabetic, chronic infection, medication)	? chest infection			
Allergies to wound care products	-			
Previous treatments used.	Dry gauze			
Pressure Relieving Equipment (e.g. pressure relieving bed, cushion)	N/A			
Wound Factors Date:	1st Sept			
Wound Classification healthy granulation epithelialisation slough black/brown necrotic tissue infected	Sloughy			
Exudate - Amount	moderate			
Odour offensive/some/none	some			
Wound Dimensions length width depth	6cm x 2cm x 2cm			
Wound Photographed?	Yes			
Pain (Site) at wound site elsewhere (specify)	wound site			
Pain (frequency) continuous/intermittent/ only at dressing changes/ at night/none	occasional			
Pain (severity) 0 = none 10 = excruciating	4			
Condition of surrounding skin (fragile, reddened, dry etc)	reddened			
Refer to CNS in Tissue Y/N Viability Date	yes - 1st Sept			
Wound Assessed by:	*D. Jones*			
Next Review date:	3rd Sept			

● *Nursing interventions* ●

Nursing care plan

Problem	Goal	Action	Rationale	Evaluation
Dehiscent surgical wound.	To promote rapid healing by 2nd intention.	(1) Clean wound by irrigation using warm saline; dry surrounding skin.	Reduces trauma to wound.	
		(2) Fill cavity with Intrasite®.	Promotes autolysis of slough and development of granulation tissue.	Weekly.
		(3) Protect surrounding skin by applying Skin Prep® to area covered by tape.	Protects skin from repeated trauma caused by removal of adhesive tape at dressing change.	Weekly.
		(4) Cover with absorbent pad and tape in place.	Absorbs exudate and provides protective barrier.	
		(5) Check dressing daily for signs of leakage; change alternate days.	Ensures optimum dressing wear time	Daily.
		(6) Record wound appearance at each dressing change; measure weekly.	Provides objective record.	Alternate days Weekly.

Date: . . . .   1 Sept. . . . . . .

Signature: . . . .   D. Jones . . . . .

The outcome of care

Mrs Briggs became much less frightened after being seen by the clinical nurse specialist. She said that she felt 'safe' in hospital. The sloughy areas in the wound debrided quickly and granulation tissue could be seen in the wound bed. The district nurse who had previously seen Mrs Briggs contacted the ward and arranged to visit and discuss arrangements for home care with the nursing staff. Mrs Briggs was discharged home 12 days after being admitted. Her wound measured 5 cm × 1 cm × 0.5 cm. It healed without further problem.

Chapter 8
Clinical Guidelines in Effective Wound Care

8.1 INTRODUCTION

Most nurses want to give their patients high-quality care. In the last few years there has been considerable emphasis placed on the importance of ensuring that clinical practice is based on research – evidence-based care. This concept has become part of the ethos that healthcare should be clinically effective (NHS Executive, 1993). The Royal College of Nursing (1996) has described clinical effectiveness as: '. . . doing the *right* thing in the *right* way at the *right* time for the *right* patient.' Research is required to identify what is 'right'.

Alongside the move to identify clinically effective practice has been the development of clinical guidelines. In turn this links to clinical audit. Research is an essential component underpinning each one. This chapter will address the issues in relation to developing clinically effective practice in wound care.

8.2 CLINICAL EFFECTIVENESS

Developing effective clinical practice involves:

- identifying current research and 'best' practice
- critically appraising the research and evaluating its value to the proposed care setting
- setting appropriate guidelines, protocols or standards
- implementing these, and changing practice where necessary
- undertaking clinical audits to measure outcomes and ensure patient care is clinically effective
- sharing this knowledge with others within the clinical care setting and elsewhere.

The NHS Executive (1998) have produced a useful document for nurses, midwives and health visitors to provide guidance on achieving effective practice. Full details are provided at the end of this chapter.

8.2.1 Searching and appraising the literature

With the advent of electronic databases, literature searches have become more sophisticated. It is no longer adequate for an individual simply to use those articles stored in the filing cabinet. They are likely to be out of date and coincide with the point of view of the individual. An electronic database can assist in rapidly identifying relevant information on a specific topic. It is also important to have access to library facilities in order to retrieve the relevant papers. Wound care research can be found in a wide range of journals as evidenced in the reference lists within this book. There are also a number of specialist journals which concentrate wholly on tissue viability or very specific types of wounds. Table 8.1 lists some examples. Hand searching these journals may also provide further information.

Table 8.1   Examples of different types of wound care journals.

General wound care journals
Advances in Wound Care
Journal of Tissue Viability*
Journal of Wound Care*
Ostomy and Wound Management

Journals that include specific types of wounds
Burns*
Journal of Burncare Rehabilitation
Journal of Hospital Infection*
Journal of Wound, Ostomy and Continence Nursing
Surgery*

---

* indicates journals that originate in the UK.

Searching the literature is very time consuming as there is a wealth of information available. Not everyone has the time or resources to undertake such a task in relation to all aspects of patient care. Systematic reviews of the literature can assist the healthcare professional by integrating existing information (Mulrow, 1994). A systematic review has been defined by Mulrow (1994) as the methodological and critical exploration, evaluation, collation and analysis of information from related research studies to draw conclusions about the variables and outcomes included in the studies. Systematic reviews generally only include randomised controlled trials as they are considered to be the best research method for measuring the effectiveness of different treatments. Within the review the results of several studies can be grouped together by means of a type of statistical analysis called meta-analysis which can give a more conclusive result than each of the studies may do on their own (Cook *et al.*, 1997b). A number of systematic reviews have been undertaken concerning wound care. Thus far, two have been published in the *Effective Health Care Bulletin* as well as in other journals.

The researchers undertaking a systematic review critically appraise the relevant research on a topic. The skill of critical appraisal should be developed by all healthcare professionals. It allows individuals to judge the value of a piece of research and whether the findings have implications for their own clinical practice. The NHS Executive (1998) suggest that critical appraisal has three stages:

- Appraisal of the study design.
- Appraisal of the conduct of the study.
- Appraisal of the outcomes of the study.

Table 8.2 lists the questions which might be asked for each of these stages.

Table 8.2   Suggested questions for critical appraisal.

Appraisal of the research design
Does the title of the study indicate what it is about?
Are the reasons for the study clearly stated?
Is there a comprehensive review of the literature?
Is the sample representative and of suitable size?
Are the data collection tools and any measurements reliable and valid?
What statistical methods have been used?

Appraisal of the conduct of the research
Was the study completed as planned?
Were the findings described adequately?
Was the analysis performed accurately?
Was statistical significance tested in the case of quantitative research?
Were the ethical issues identified and managed appropriately?

Appraisal of the outcomes of the research
What is the clinical significance of the findings of the study?
How have the hypotheses been interpreted (when assessing quantitative research)?
Are the conclusions drawn by the researcher(s) justified?
Do the findings compare with those from other studies?
Can the findings be applied to your own patients?

Based on NHS Executive (1998).

8.2.2 Developing clinical guidelines

Clinical guidelines have been defined as 'systematically developed statements to assist practitioner and patient decisions about appropriate health care for specific clinical circumstances' (Field & Lohr, 1992). The purpose of clinical guidelines is to improve the clinical effectiveness of healthcare by identifying good practice and the desired outcomes of clinical care (Scottish Intercollegiate Guidelines Network (SIGN), 1995). Guidelines may be developed on an international, national or local level; however, they are most effective when they are adapted for local use (Effective Health Care, 1994).

Generally, guidelines consist of a series of statements about a particular topic with a rationale for each statement. The rationale relates to the evidence, usually obtained from systematic reviews, underpinning the statement. Many guidelines use a hierarchy to measure the quality of the evidence that they use and then grade the recommendations within the guideline. SIGN (1995) uses this approach. For example, within the hierarchy of evidence Level 1b indicates evidence obtained from at least one randomised controlled trial; a statement based on this evidence would be graded as a Grade A statement. Table 8.3 shows the grading system used in the European Pressure Ulcer Advisory Panel guidelines for pressure sore prevention.

Preparation and publication of a guideline is not enough to ensure that it is implemented. Any national guideline tends to be written in broad terms. It needs to be adapted to include more operational detail for local use and may include policies and protocols. The development team should be multidisciplinary reflecting all key personnel including representatives from purchasing authorities (Effective Health

Table 8.3 The grading of recommendations within the European Pressure Ulcer Advisory Panel guidelines on pressure ulcer prevention.

Grade A
Requires the results of two or more randomised controlled clinical trials on pressure ulcers in humans to provide support.

Grade B
Requires the results of two or more controlled clinical trials on pressure ulcers in humans to provide support, or, where appropriate, results of two or more controlled trials in an animal model to provide indirect support.

Grade C
This grade requires one or more of the following:

(1) results of one controlled trial
(2) results of at least two case series/descriptive studies on pressure ulcers in humans
(3) expert opinion.

European Pressure Ulcer Advisory Panel (1998).

Care, 1994). Effective implementation is best achieved by means of active education programmes for those whose work is affected by the guideline (Onion *et al.*, 1996). Where possible, it is beneficial to introduce prompts into patient records which remind the professional to follow the guideline (Effective Health Care, 1994). It is important to monitor patient outcomes to determine any health benefits from introducing the guideline. This may be achieved by the audit cycle.

8.2.3 The clinical audit cycle

Audit has been defined as 'a clinically led initiative which seeks to improve the quality and outcome of patient care through structured peer review whereby clinicians examine their practices and results against agreed explicit standards and modify their practice where indicated' (NHS Executive, 1996). Burnett and Winyard (1998) suggest that clinical audit is at the heart of clinical effectiveness. The audit process is cyclical as shown in Figure 8.1.

One of the benefits of audit is that it can be used to measure the outcomes of everyday practice to provide baseline information before introducing clinical guidelines. A repeat of the audit enables the guideline team to monitor any health gains associated with the implementation of more effective practice as well as monitoring whether the guidelines are being adhered to. Staff are likely to be more willing to maintain adherence to guidelines if they can see a beneficial outcome. Providing information for staff about performance levels is an essential aspect of the audit process.

8.2.4 Disseminating audit findings

As well as sharing audit results with those directly involved, it is important to discuss them with a wider audience. This may be in the form of a report for the executive

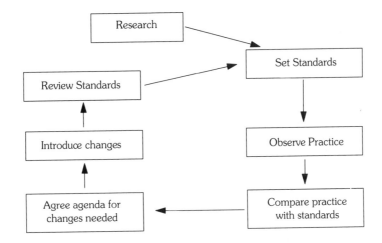

Fig. 8.1   The audit cycle.

board of a hospital trust or the local purchasing authority, or it may be a conference presentation or a publication. There are a number of benefits:

- Internal dissemination allows other areas in the organisation to benefit from the audit findings.
- Others working in similar clinical areas can apply the lessons learned from the audit.
- The individuals concerned can develop skills in writing and undertaking presentations

8.3 CLINICALLY EFFECTIVE WOUND CARE

Within wound care there are three topics which have been considered to be good indicators of the quality of healthcare provision: pressure sore prevention; the management of venous leg ulcers; and surgical wound infection rates. They will be used as examples of the implementation of clinically effective wound care.

8.3.1 Appraising the literature on wound care

The literature pertaining to all aspects of wound care is huge, many examples have been given in other chapters of this book. It is, therefore, important for the nurse to be aware of how to identify both the strengths and the weaknesses of the wound care evidence.

Early studies of modern dressings tended to compare them with gauze. As the differences between the two groups were so great only relatively small numbers of patients were needed in a study. However, the differences are much smaller when comparing two modern products and therefore much larger numbers are needed. It may be difficult for one centre to recruit sufficient patients, so several centres may be required. This may introduce other variables if there are differences in local management patterns (Freak, 1995). High-quality research will indicate that it has addressed this problem by using a power calculation to identify the required sample size and addressing the issue of standardisation between centres.

Another issue to consider when appraising the wound care literature is endpoints. In other words at what point a patient should be considered to have completed a study. Freak (1995) suggests that complete healing is not always the most suitable endpoint. Certainly a study of debridement would require a different endpoint – a granulating wound. Six weeks may be a reasonable length of time to assess the efficacy of a dressing on a pressure sore but the time may need to be longer for leg ulcer studies. Nelson (1998) suggests that healing rates for leg ulcers should be measured at intervals over a period of probably more than 12 weeks.

Systematic reviews take these factors into consideration when appraising the literature. The systematic reviews of pressure sore prevention and treatment, and of the use of compression for venous ulceration, have been widely used, including in Chapter 5 of this book. There are a number of systematic reviews in relation to wound care in preparation (Fletcher et al. (1997). Once all these reviews have been published it will help to clarify the areas where further research is required.

8.3.2 Guidelines in wound care

Developing guidelines is costly (Nelson, 1997). It makes economic sense for trusts to utilise guidelines developed at a national level where possible and then adapt them to local use. There are a great number of guidelines available for both pressure sores and leg ulcers. Many have been published in the wound care literature. Since they are generally based on the same research there are many similarities between them. At present there is insufficient high-quality research to provide all Grade A recommendations in guidelines for either pressure sores or leg ulcers. For example, the European Pressure Ulcer Advisory Panel prevention guidelines (European Pressure Ulcer Advisory Panel, 1998) comprise 26 statements of which one is Grade A, six are Grade B and the remaining 19 are Grade C. Cook et al. (1997a) suggest that where the evidence supporting a guideline is not strong, the impact of implementation needs to be rigorously audited.

8.3.3 Auditing clinical practice

Audit provides data both for initial baseline information and to measure the outcomes of guideline implementation. In many instances this information is obtained by means of prevalence surveys and incidence monitoring. This is particularly true of pressure sores where there has been much debate on the most effective methods for collecting this information and on its value.

Prevalence can be defined as:

'The number of persons with a specific disease or condition as a proportion of a given population measured at a specific point in time.' (Dealey, 1997)

Whereas incidence is defined as:

'The number of people developing a specific condition as a proportion of the local population measured over a period of time.' (Dealey, 1997)

An example of a baseline pressure sore audit is one undertaken in France by Barrois *et al.* (1997). They found an overall prevalence of 8.7% and documented in considerable detail the characteristics of pressure sores in France. This provided a very informative baseline prior to introducing a range of prevention strategies. Incidence rates are often used to evaluate the effectiveness of prevention policies. Data collection for incidence measurement is more complicated than for prevalence surveys and subject to inaccuracies (Bridel *et al.*, 1996). However, Dealey (1997) suggests that the main benefit of incidence is to demonstrate improvements over time.

Lindholm *et al.* (1998) and Dealey (1998) undertook prevalence surveys of leg ulceration prior to instigating education and training and the implementation of management guidelines. Audit of the effectiveness of this strategy concentrated on changes in practice, nursing knowledge and healing rates (Dealey, 1998). Feedback of the results to the staff provided encouragement that adherence to the guidelines was ensuring increased healing rates. Stevens *et al.* (1997) also used healing rates to monitor the outcomes of a project establishing leg ulcer guidelines within two acute hospitals and the surrounding community. Over time they were also able to measure recurrence rates and compare them favourably with the rate from another study previously reported in the literature.

Audit of surgical wounds is usually undertaken as a surveillance of wound infection rates. This may be in the form of either prevalence or incidence. Prevalence surveys have been used in national surveys to provide a snapshot of the situation (Briggs, 1996). Incidence rates can be used to monitor the performance of individual surgeons. Frequently this type of surveillance measures the incidence of surgical wound infection (SWI) in clean surgery. Incidence may be used with case-control studies or with cohort studies. Case-control studies retrospectively compare a group of patients with SWI with a group of patients without SWI in order to determine any risk factors associated with SWI. Cohort studies are prospective and follow a group of patients over time to see who develops a SWI. Potential risk factors are determined at the beginning of the studies and then monitored for the outcome. For example, in their ten-year study Cruse and Foord (1980) considered diabetes to be a potential risk factor and so monitored the clean wound infection rate for diabetic patients and found it to be considerably higher than for patients without diabetes. The findings from this type of audit can be used to improve patient care.

8.4 CONCLUSIONS

At present the quality of the evidence available to support clinically effective wound care is very variable. Systematic reviews can be used to determine the gaps so that future research can be directed to the area where it is most needed.

FURTHER INFORMATION

NHS Executive (1998) *Achieving Effective Practice: A Clinical Effectiveness and Research Information Pack for Nurses, Midwives and Health Visitors*. Department of Health, London. Code No. 13902 NUR 10k 2P SEPT 98 (MPS). For copies call the NHS Response line 0541 555455.

REFERENCES

Barrois, B., Allaert, F., Urbinelli, R., Colin, D. (1997) National survey in France: pressure sores in hospital institutions in 1994, in (eds) Cherry, G.W., Gottrup, F., Lawrence, J.C., Moffat, C.J., Turner, T.D., *Proceedings of the 5th European Conference on Advances in Wound Management*. Macmillan Magazines Ltd, London.

Bridel, J., Banks, S., Mitton, C. (1996) The admission prevalence and hospital-acquired incidence of pressure sores within a large teaching hospital during April 1994 to March 1995, in (eds) Cherry, G.W., Gottrup, F., Lawrence, J.C., Moffat, C.J., Turner, T.D., *Proceedings of the 5th European Conference on Advances in Wound Management*. Macmillan Magazines Ltd, London.

Briggs, M. (1996) Epidemiological methods in the study of surgical wound infection. *Journal of Wound Care*, **5** (4), 186–191.

Burnett, A.C., Winyard, G. (1998) Clinical audit at the heart of clinical effectiveness. *Journal of Quality and Clinical Practice*, **18** (1), 3–19.

Cook, D.J., Greengold, N.L., Ellrodt, A.G., Weingarten, S.R. (1997a) The relation between systematic reviews and practice guidelines. *Annals of Internal Medicine*, **127** (3), 210–216.

Cook, D.J., Mulrow, C.D., Haynes, R.B. (1997b) Systematic reviews: synthesis of best evidence for clinical decisions. *Annals of Internal Medicine*, **126** (5), 376–380.

Cruse, P.J.E., Foord, R. (1980) The epidemiology of wound infection: a 10-year prospective study of 62,939 wounds. *Surgical Clinics of North America*, **60**, 27–40.

Dealey, C. (1997) *Managing Pressure Sore Prevention*. Mark Allen Publishing Ltd, Salisbury.

Dealey, C. (1998) The importance of education in effecting change in leg ulcer management, in (eds) Leaper, D., Dealey, C., Franks, P.J., Hofman, D., Moffatt, C.J., *Proceedings of the 7th European Conference on Advances in Wound Management*. EMAP Healthcare Ltd, London.

Effective Health Care (1994) Implementing clinical practice guidelines. *Effective Health Care Bulletin no. 8*. University of Leeds, Leeds.

European Pressure Ulcer Advisory Panel (1998) A policy statement on the prevention of pressure ulcers from the European Pressure Ulcer Advisory Panel. *British Journal of Nursing*, **7** (15), 888–890.

Field, M.J., Lohr, K.N. (1992) *Guidelines for Clinical Practice: From Development to Use*. National Academy Press, Washington, DC.

Fletcher, A., Cullum, N., Sheldon, T., Song, F. (1997) Identifying evidence-based wound care: systematic reviews and the Cochrane collaboration, in (eds) Leaper, D.J., Cherry, G.W., Dealey, C., Lawrence, J.C., Turner, T.D., *Proceedings of the 6th European Conference on Advances in Wound Management*. Macmillan Magazines Ltd, London.

Freak, L. (1995) Evaluating clinical trials. *Journal of Wound Care*, **4** (3), 114–116.

Lindholm, C., Tammelin, A., Bergsten, A., Berglund, E. (1998) The Uppsala experience: implications for developing educational strategies, in (eds) Leaper, D., Dealey, C., Franks, P.J., Hofman, D., Moffatt, C.J., *Proceedings of the 7th European Conference on Advances in Wound Management.* EMAP Healthcare Ltd, London.

Mulrow, C.D. (1994) Rationale for systematic reviews. *British Medical Journal,* **309** (6954), 597–599.

Nelson E.A. (1997) Clinical guidelines. *Journal of Wound Care,* **6** (8), 402–404.

Nelson, E.A. (1998) The evidence in support of compression bandaging. *Journal of Wound Care,* **7** (3), 148–150.

NHS Executive (1993) *Improving Clinical Effectiveness, EL(93)115.* Department of Health, Leeds.

NHS Executive (1996) *Clinical Audit in the NHS. Using Clinical Audit in the NHS: A Position Statement.* Department of Health, Leeds.

NHS Executive (1998) *Achieving Effective Practice: A Clinical Effectiveness and Research Information Pack for Nurses, Midwives and Health Visitors.* Department of Health, London.

Onion, C.W., Dutton, C.E., Walley, T., Turnball, C.J., Dunne, W.T., Buchan, I.E. (1996) Local clinical guidelines: description and evaluation of a participative method for their development and evaluation. *Family Practice,* **13** (1), 28–34.

Royal College of Nursing (1996) *Clinical Effectiveness.* RCN, London.

Scottish Intercollegiate Guidelines Network (SIGN) (1995) *Clinical Guidelines: Criteria for Appraisal for National Use.* Scottish Intercollegiate Guidelines Network, Edinburgh.

Stevens, J., Franks, P.J., Harrington, M. (1997) A community/hospital leg ulcer service. *Journal of Wound Care,* **6** (2), 62–68.

Chapter 9
Conclusions

9.1 INTRODUCTION

This chapter seeks to address several issues related to wound care which do not fall readily into the other chapters. Some of the issues may be described as contentious and although it is intended to provide a rounded view of each specific issue, the conclusions are those of the author.

9.2 THE COST OF HEALING

The emphasis so far in this book has been to consider wound care without reference to the cost involved. Much attention has been given to the modern products and the research supporting their use. Although there is little doubt as to the efficacy of these dressings, their use is by no means universal. One of the reasons may be cost.

Generally, when a product is chosen to dress a wound, little attention is paid to the cost of the materials being used. However, it is true that the *choice* of dressings is often limited because of cost. The decision regarding the particular products from which to choose may be made by non-clinicians without reference to the user. There is an increasing interest in cost-effective care and the use of audit. Nurses need to become aware of the cost of the care they give so that they can argue their case effectively for quality of care. This should not just be limited to the basic cost of dressings – although it does have a part to play – but should also look at the wider issues.

9.2.1 The cost of materials

Many of the second generation dressings are considerably more expensive than the traditional dressings that they have replaced. A piece of gauze costs a few pence, whereas the new dressings can cost in the region of £2–£3 for a 10 × 10 cm size. Inevitably, there has been resistance to their introduction on grounds of cost. But the major advantage of these dressings is that they do not require daily changing and that they may well speed up the healing process.

Several studies have looked at the costs associated with using a modern product compared with traditional dressings. Ohlsson *et al.* (1994) compared the use of hydrocolloid dressings with saline-soaked gauze for community leg ulcer patients. They found the material costs to be similar. However, when the nursing time and the travel costs were considered they found the mean cost for patients in the gauze group was 4126 Swedish Kronor and for patients in the hydrocolloid group it was 1565 Swedish Kronor.

Cannavo *et al.* (1998) compared three types of dressing: an alginate, sodium hypochlorite soaked ribbon gauze, and a combined dressing pad for use on dehiscent surgical abdominal wounds. The alginate dressing was the most expensive when considered on a per dressing basis. However, when the costs for material use and nursing time were calculated then the sodium hypochlorite soaked ribbon gauze was found to be considerably more expensive – A\$19.36 a day compared with A\$15.25 a day for the alginate. A similar study by Ricci *et al.* (1998) compared foam stents with iodine-soaked gauze in surgical cavities. Although they did not do actual costings, they measured the number of dressings used and found that six patients required 20 foam stents compared with 868 gauze soaks required for the other six patients.

9.2.2 The cost to the hospital

The cost to the hospital has to be considered in terms of delayed healing or complications delaying recovery. Two areas which can be considered are pressure sores and surgical wound infection. Much work has been undertaken on prevention and management of pressure sores. One classic study by Hibbs (1988) calculated the cost of treating a patient with a Grade 4 pressure sore which developed as a complication of hip surgery. Every cost was included, such as nursing time, catering costs, domestic services, X-rays and so on. The patient was in hospital for 180 days at a total cost of £25 905.58. Further calculations showed that the money spent treating this patient would have paid for 20 standard cases. In the time that the bed was 'blocked' a further 16 hip or knee replacements could have been undertaken.

Xakellis *et al.* (1998) calculated the costs of pressure sore incidence in a long-term care facility before and after introducing a pressure sore prevention protocol. They found a drop in the incidence rate from 23% to 5% after the introduction of the protocol. The mean cost of pressure sore prevention and treatment was \$113 ± \$345 per subject before the protocol was introduced and \$113 ± \$157 per subject after it was in use. This was a significant reduction of both incidence and costs.

With the increase in litigation, some patients have taken action against health authorities and trusts for the development of a pressure sore. Tingle (1997) has reviewed some of the court cases arising from pressure sore litigation where sums ranging from £3500 to £12 500 were awarded to the plaintiffs.

Surgical audit is a useful way of counting the cost of wound infection post-operatively. Several studies have considered the costs associated with surgical wound infection (SWI). DiPiro *et al.* (1998) monitored 288 906 surgical patients of whom 11.9% developed an infection. They found the mean length of stay for those with a SWI was 14 days compared with four days for those without infection. Zoutman *et al.* (1998) monitored all the costs associated with SWI in one hospital over a 12-month period. The total costs for 108 patients with SWI was \$321 533. These patients required a mean of 10.2 days extended length of stay.

9.2.3 The cost to the patient

For the many people suffering from chronic wounds there is no way their pain and suffering can be quantified, neither can the effect it has on their quality of life. Leg ulcers are classic examples. Chase *et al.* (1997) undertook a study of patients' experiences of leg ulceration in an ambulatory leg ulcer clinic. They found that for most patients the leg ulcers became a major part of their life, restricting their mobility and causing them to live with chronic pain. Several patients lost their jobs as a consequence of the ulcer. They also felt powerless to control the slow rate of healing, and subsequent recurrence was seen as inevitable.

Social isolation is another aspect of unrecognised cost to many people. Many patients are very conscious of the odour from their wounds and so refuse to go out. For others, sadly, the nurse dressing their ulcer may be the only real contact with the outside world. One small study found that those patients with the lowest number of social contacts were those whose ulcers recurred within a six-month period (Wise, 1986). So, for those people, the cost of healing was actually social isolation.

The cost to a younger person is not only in pain, but also in loss of earnings which may cause considerable hardship. It may also affect future employment. There is disruption of family life; even visiting hospital may be difficult for the partner if there are young children in the family. It should also be remembered that there is still a mortality risk from postoperative complications following any surgery. DiPiro *et al.* (1998) found that the in-hospital mortality rate was 14.5% of infected patients compared with 1.8% for non-infected patients.

9.2.4 The cost to the community

The idea that poorly healing wounds have a cost to the community is one that has not really been explored. An infected wound, as well as causing unnecessary pain and suffering to the patient and delaying discharge from hospital, also means a loss of productive work. A person's labour not only earns money for the labourer, but is also a benefit to the community in terms of goods produced or services rendered and taxes paid. If this is lost through incapacity, then the cost is not only that of the loss but also the cost of sickness benefit. This is not to say that such rights should not be available, indeed they should, but their cost should be recognised.

9.2.5 Conclusions

So what is the true cost of healing? It is obvious that there is no easy answer. It is most certainly more than comparing the cost of a piece of gauze with that of a film dressing. The *Code of Conduct* exhorts nurses always to act so as to 'serve the interests of society, and above all to safeguard the interests of individual patients and clients' (UKCC, 1992a). This surely means that quality of care is paramount.

As the use of various types of audit becomes a more frequent part of hospital life, this provides an opportunity to demonstrate that quality of care can be cost effective. There is a case for adequate prevention of both pressure sores and post-operative wound infection as well as appropriate wound management. Nurses should see that part of their role is to ensure that the hospital does the patient no harm.

9.3 NURSES AND THEIR ROLE IN WOUND CARE

Nurses have an important role to play in wound management and need to be aware of their responsibilities. Obviously this role must be seen in the context of the multidisciplinary team, as wounds cannot be seen in isolation from the rest of the body. Many different medical specialities are also involved in wound care, so the constituent members may vary according to the needs of the patient. In many areas, multidisciplinary teams are preparing policies in relation to wound management and pressure sore prevention. Such efforts are to be applauded as they can make major improvements to the standards of patient care.

9.3.1 Accountability

The UKCC *Code of Professional Conduct* (UKCC, 1992a) states that nurses are accountable for their actions. Ralph (1990) suggested that professional account-ability is an obligation on practitioners that binds them to a code of conduct which is based on the expectations of society that individual nurses will use their own dis-cretion and skill to safeguard their patients and act in every way to uphold pro-fessional standards. It must also be emphasised that the prescriptive authority that doctors have over nurses does not absolve nurses from the consequences of their actions. If a doctor prescribes an inappropriate dosage of a drug which is then administered by a nurse, the nurse also has to accept some responsibility and be held to account for individual actions.

As well as being accountable professionally to the UKCC, nurses also have a duty of care to their patients. Failure to take due care which results in harm to a patient is negligence (Young, 1995). Reasonable care as applied to the medical profession has been defined as the standard of a reasonably skilled and experi-enced doctor as accepted by a reasonable body of doctors skilled in that parti-cular art. This is called the Bolam test as it is taken from the case of Bolam v. Friern Hospital Management Committee (1957) and it can be applied to any professional (UKCC, 1996).

The UKCC (1996) produced a document entitled *Guidelines for Professional Practice* to give guidance on the application of the statements within the *Code of Conduct*. This document is divided into a number of sections most of which have relevance to wound care.

The sections on patient advocacy, communicating, truthfulness and consent will be considered together. Patients have the right to choose whether to accept or refuse care. In order to make an informed decision a patient needs to know all the relevant facts. Communication is extremely important and involves active listening as well as speaking. Good record keeping is also essential. Seeking consent from a patient may mean making compromises if a patient is not willing to accept all the aspects of a particular treatment. For example, if a patient is not prepared to tolerate high compression for leg ulceration, for whatever reason, an acceptable alternative should be found.

A further responsibility the nurse has is that of highlighting inadequate provision of patient care. Inadequate provision of care is seen as negligence in law (Livesley & Simpson, 1989). This can be related to matters such as an insufficient supply of pressure-relieving equipment. The nurse should be prepared to make representation to a higher authority and, most importantly, maintain accurate records of what the consequences might be for the patient without the equipment.

One section in the document discusses the importance of nurses working with other professionals and agencies in a spirit of co-operation and collaboration. The concept of working in teams has improved over recent years, but problems can still arise. Very often they may be related to issues concerning decision making in wound care.

9.3.2 Decision making in wound care

Any discussion of the role of the nurse in wound care has to consider the relationship between medicine and nursing. There is considerable overlap between the knowledge base of the two professions. Nurses and doctors can be described as key players in the field of treatment and care of patients (RCN, 1990). There is no clear-cut division of responsibility between the two. Instead there is a need to work in harmony together.

Essential aspects of wound management are assessment of the wound and planning appropriate treatment. There has been much discussion about who should make these decisions – the nurse or the doctor. Kulkarni and Philbin (1993) surveyed doctors, nurses and therapists to assess awareness of pressure sore prevention strategies. They found that nurses had the greatest knowledge of the subject and that doctors were not particularly interested in it.

A very small study was carried out by Chandler (1990) who interviewed both nurses and doctors on two surgical wards. She found that the nurses had a far greater awareness of current research and modern products than did the doctors. However, despite this, they still relied on the doctors to determine the dressing to be used. The doctors' choice was mostly based on preference or habit.

Gwyther (1988) questioned 85 student and qualified nurses regarding wound care practices. One question addressed the issue of decision making. Some 83.5% felt it was a sister or staff nurse who chose the dressing to be used whereas 45.9% suggested that the decision was made by a doctor. No specific type of wound was indicated in the question. It should also be noted that 92.9% of the respondents said that they had been taught about wound assessment.

Flanagan (1992) interviewed 24 qualified nurses about their views on wound care. They were all aware of the clinical factors which influence dressing selection. However, they tended to be more interested in discussing the influence of the medical staff on dressing choice. Many expressed anxiety about the differences of opinion which arose between the two disciplines. They also described the types of manipulative behaviour that could be displayed by both nurses and doctors. There seemed to be some inconsistency between specialist areas. Nurses in medical areas, intensive care units, and accident and emergency departments were more likely to be able to select treatments than those working in surgical wards.

These studies highlight several issues:

(1) Nurses seem to make most of the decisions in relation to pressure sore management, possibly because pressure sores have traditionally been seen as a nursing problem.
(2) Surgeons inevitably seem to have a greater interest in choosing dressings, seeing the surgical wound as their responsibility.
(3) Although research into wound management has had a high profile in nursing journals, this has not been so in medical journals.
(4) The fact that nurses actually carry out the dressing change means that they have more confidence in the use of dressings and their mode of action than do their medical colleagues. This is particularly of relevance when using interactive wound management products.
(5) There are many anecdotal reports of conflict between nurses and doctors over what constitutes an appropriate dressing. However, they are not as frequent as they used to be.

Many nurses believe that they should automatically have the right to choose a suitable dressing for the patient, and in practice many actually make that decision. In short, having the right to select a dressing can be seen as one aspect of autonomy, or freedom to act. Vaughan (1989) suggests that autonomy is not complete freedom, but 'freedom to act within the bounds of competence, which are in turn confined by the boundaries of knowledge'. Nurses should not be seeking such autonomy unless they have sufficient knowledge and competence for the task in hand. The discussions related to the right of the community nurse to prescribe a limited range of products has heightened awareness of the importance of education and training. Autonomy and accountability carry responsibilities. The document *The Scope of Professional Practice* (UKCC, 1992b) states the principles that must be maintained within nursing practice. They include honestly acknowledging the limits of personal skills and knowledge as well as ensuring that any extension of professional practice always conforms to the *Code of Practice*.

It must always be remembered that the wound cannot be treated in isolation; it is, after all, attached to a patient. Medical intervention may well be needed for effective treatment. For example, vascular surgery may be necessary for ischaemic ulcers to heal. There are many examples where nursing and medicine complement each other and it is important for each discipline to have respect for the other.

9.3.3 The nursing process

Assessment and planning

Assessment of the patient and the wound should be carried out and recorded in a methodical manner. In 1998, the UKCC produced the document *Guidelines for Records and Record Keeping* to provide advice on both the professional and legal responsibilities of nurses. Records are perceived to be an integral and essential part of care allowing good communication between professionals. Assessment may reveal the need to involve other members of the multidisciplinary team in the care of the patient. In the case of patients at risk of developing pressure sores or those already suffering from them, specialist equipment may be required. The nurse has a major role in planning these aspects of care and in co-ordinating the input from other members of the team. Thus, a coherent strategy can be established which maximises wound healing.

Implementation

Although there may be dispute over who assesses a wound and plans the care, there is none over implementation of the plan. The vast majority of wounds are dressed by nurses. Applying a dressing which is both comfortable and remains in place requires a degree of manual dexterity. Experience is also of considerable importance. An understanding of the action of the interactive wound management products is also necessary when removing the old dressing.

Evaluation

At each dressing change the nurse should monitor the progress of the wound and the effectiveness of the dressing. Evaluation is an ongoing process. Part of evaluation must also be documentation and communication with others. Effective documentation will record the size and appearance of the wound. Any changes need to be communicated to others as part of the exchange of information about patient progress.

9.3.4 Education

Another aspect of the role of the nurse in wound care is providing education to others. Patient education is important to enhance compliance and understanding of different aspects of care. Nurses may also require information about any aspect of wound management. There is also a need to provide education for medical students and junior doctors. A survey by Bennet (1992) of medical undergraduate teaching on chronic wound care found that tuition ranged from 0 to 35.5 hours. Since this survey there has been a reorganisation of medical training resulting in the development of special study modules as well as core modules. Several medical schools now include wound management topics within both types of module (Davis, 1996). Practical experience will still be gained on the wards. It is already recognised that nurses teach junior doctors a great deal when they are first qualified; wound management is yet another topic which requires consideration.

9.3.5 Nurse specialist in wound care

A new nursing speciality developed in the late 1980s – that of the specialist in wound care. Flanagan (1997) identified 110 nurse specialists in the UK. The precise number is difficult to determine as there is no formal register and the precise title may vary. The most frequently used are 'clinical nurse specialist in tissue viability' and 'wound care specialist'. Flanagan (1997) found that 90% had been appointed to a new post, demonstrating the recent emergence of this speciality. Education is an essential prerequisite for the recognition of any speciality. Fletcher (1998) found that there are a variety of courses available within the UK. They comprise short courses at diploma level as well as degree and masters level programmes. Unfortunately, there is considerable variation in both cost and geographical spread.

A major aspect of the role of the specialist is in providing expert advice on the management and prevention of wounds of all types. As well as having a good understanding of the range of wound management products, many of these specialist nurses are able to provide guidance on the selection of pressure-relieving mattresses and beds. The specialist may be called upon to negotiate with others in relation to the care that is needed for particular patients. Much of the clinical care that is given provides ideal teaching opportunities on a one-to-one basis. A number of nurse specialists are involved in wider teaching at study days and conferences. Many hospitals and units are developing policies to cover standards in wound management, formularies of wound management products and strategies for pressure sore prevention. The wound care specialist can play an integral role in the development and implementation of such policies.

Many nurse specialists are involved in research in a whole range of aspects of wound healing. They include pressure sore prevalence and incidence monitoring, surveys of equipment, surveys of nursing practice, evaluations of products and equipment as well as aspects of cell biology.

Although the role of the clinical nurse specialist can be challenging and very rewarding there is also the potential for burnout (Flanagan, 1996). She describes some of the difficulties that the clinical nurse specialist may face. They include unrealistic objectives or targets, role ambiguity, responsibilities across large geographical areas or multiple sites, constant pressure to reduce the cost of the tissue viability service and often insufficient resources with limited professional support. Despite the constraints the role of the clinical nurse specialist still presents the post-holder with considerable opportunities to enhance nursing practice.

9.3.6 Conclusions

Nurses have an important role to play in wound care as summarised in Fig. 9.1. However, they do not work in isolation and optimal care can only be provided in the context of the multidisciplinary team. Ultimately, nurses are accountable to their patients. In order to provide the highest standards of care, nurses should ensure that they are aware of recent developments in the field and of their implications for practice.

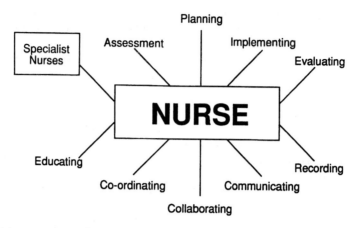

Fig. 9.1 The role of the nurse in wound care.

REFERENCES

Bennet, G. (1992) Medical undergraduate teaching in chronic wound care (a survey). *Journal of Tissue Viability*, **2** (2), 50–51.

Cannavo, M., Fairbrother, G., Owen, D., Ingle, J., Lumley, T. (1998) A comparison of dressings in the management of surgical abdominal wounds. *Journal of Wound Care*, **7** (2), 57–62.

Chandler, S. (1990) Wound management in surgical wards. *Nursing Times*, **86** (27), 54.

Chase, S.K., Melloni, M., Savage, A. (1997) A forever healing: the lived experience of leg ulcer disease. *Journal of Vascular Nursing*, **15**, 73–78.

Davis, M. (1996) Wound-care training in medical education. *Journal of Wound Care*, **5** (6), 286–287.

DiPiro, J.T., Martindale, R.G., Bakst, A., Vacani, P.F., Watson, P., Miller, M.T. (1998) Infection in surgical wounds: effects on mortality, hospitalisation and postdischarge care. *American Journal of Health System Pharmacy*, **55** (8), 777–781.

Flanagan, M. (1992) Outside influences. *Nursing Times*, **88** (36), 72–78.

Flanagan, M. (1996) The role of the clinical nurse specialist in tissue viability. *British Journal of Nursing*, **5** (11), 676–681.

Flanagan, M. (1997) A profile of the nurse specialist in tissue viability in the UK. *Journal of Wound Care*, **6** (2), 85–87.

Fletcher, J. (1998) A survey of courses available that are relevant to the field of tissue viability, in (eds) Leaper, D., Dealey, C., Franks, P.J., Hofman, D., Moffatt, C., *Proceedings of the 7th European Conference on Advances in Wound Management*. EMAP Healthcare Ltd, London.

Gwyther, J. (1988) Skilled dressing. *Nursing Times*, **84** (19), 60–61.

Hibbs, P. (1988) *Pressure Area Care for the City & Hackney Health Authority*. City & Hackney Health Authority, London.

Kulkarni, J., Philbin, M. (1993) Pressure sore awareness in a university teaching hospital. *Journal of Tissue Viability*, **3** (3), 77–79.

Livesley, B., Simpson, G. (1989) The hard cost of soft sores. *Health Service Journal*, **99** (5138), 231.

Ohlsson, P., Larsson, K., Lindholm, C., Moller, M. (1994) A cost-effectiveness study of leg ulcer treatment in primary care. Comparison of saline-gauze and hydrocolloid treatment in a prospective, randomised study. *Scandinavian Journal of Primary Health Care*, **12** (4), 295–299.

Ralph, C. (1990) Nursing management and leadership – the challenge, in (eds) Jolley, M., Allan, P., *Current Issues in Nursing Development*. Croom Helm, Beckenham, Kent.

Ricci, E., Aloesio, R., Cassino, R., Ferraris, C., Gorrino, S., Anselmetti, G. (1998) Foam dressing versus gauze soaks in the treatment of surgical wounds healing by secondary intention, in (eds) Leaper, D., Cherry, G., Cockbill, S., Dealey, C., Flanagan, M., Hofman, D., *et al.*, *Proceedings of the EWMA/Journal of Wound Care Spring Meeting*. Macmillan Magazines Ltd, London.

Royal College of Nursing (1990) *Accountability in Nursing – A Discussion Document*. RCN, London.

Tingle, J. (1997) Pressure sores: counting the legal cost of nursing neglect. *British Journal of Nursing*, **6** (13), 757–758.

United Kingdom Central Council for Nursing, Midwifery and Health Visiting (1992a) *The Code of Professional Conduct for the Nurse, Midwife and Health Visitor*. UKCC, London.

United Kingdom Central Council for Nursing, Midwifery and Health Visiting (1992b) *The Scope of Professional Practice*. UKCC, London.

United Kingdom Central Council for Nursing, Midwifery and Health Visiting (1996) *Guidelines for Professional Practice*. UKCC, London.

United Kingdom Central Council for Nursing, Midwifery and Health Visiting (1998) *Guidelines for Records and Record Keeping*. UKCC, London.

Vaughan, B. (1989) Autonomy and accountability. *Nursing Times*, **85** (3), 54–55.

Wise, A. (1986) The social ulcer. *Nursing Times*, **82** (21), 47–49.

Xakellis, G.C., Frantz, R.A., Lewis, A., Harvey, P. (1998) Cost-effectiveness of an intensive pressure ulcer prevention protocol in long-term care. *Advances in Wound Care*, **11** (1), 22–29.

Young, A. (1995) Negligence. *British Journal of Nursing*, **4** (2), 119.

Zoutman, D., McDonald, S., Vethanayagan, D. (1998) Total and attributable costs of surgical-wound infections at a Canadian tertiary-care centre. *Infection Control and Hospital Epidemiology*, **19** (4), 254–259.

Glossary

Angiogenesis	The growth of new blood vessels.
Autolysis	Breaking down of devitalised tissue.
Cellulitis	Inflammation of subcutaneous tissue with localised oedema.
Colonisation	The presence of bacteria on the wound surface.
Contraction	The process where the surface area of the open wound is reduced. This occurs during the process of reconstruction in the healing wound.
Contractures	Fibrosis in the maturing scar tissue which results in shortening of the scar.
Debridement	Removal of necrotic or devitalised tissue from the wound either surgically, chemically or by autolysis.
Dehiscence	The splitting open of a closed wound.
Diapedesis	The method by which white cells move.
Eschar	The thick, hard necrotic scab covering a wound.
Exudate	Fluid which collects in a wound due to increased capillary permeability.
Granulation tissue	Fragile connective tissue containing new collagen, fibroblasts and capillary loops. Often described as 'beefy' red in colour.
Ischaemia	Localised deficiency of the blood supply.
Maceration	Softening of tissue, often around wound margins. It is associated with excessive moisture and is susceptible to breakdown.
Necrosis	Death of a portion of tissue.
Phagocytosis	The engulfing and destruction of bacteria, foreign bodies and necrotic tissue.
Tensile strength	The maximum pressure that can be applied to a wound without causing it to break apart.

Index